Fresh Medicine

Fresh Medicine

How to Fix Reform and Build a
Sustainable Health Care System

PHILIP BREDESEN

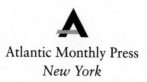

Atlantic Monthly Press
New York

Published simultaneously in Canada
Printed in the United States of America

FIRST EDITION

ISBN-13: 978-0-8021-1938-4

Atlantic Monthly Press
an imprint of Grove/Atlantic, Inc.
841 Broadway
New York, NY 10003

Distributed by Publishers Group West

www.groveatlantic.com

10 11 12 13   10 9 8 7 6 5 4 3 2 1

Contents

Fresh Medicine

Introduction

This book has a simple thesis.

- Health care in America is broken. Its costs are unsustainable and endanger our nation; its quality inconsistent.
- The underlying structure of our health care system—the insurance paradigm for payment and the uncoordinated cottage industries of providers—is obsolete.
- Congress and the Obama Administration have just added over thirty million more people into an obsolete and broken system and done little to address the underlying problems; in multiple ways they've made them worse.
- The American health care system needs a new set of principles. They should be:
  - the highest quality in the world
  - able to keep costs under control, realistic in comparison to other priorities, and fairly apportioned
  - paid for
  - universal, with a basic level of care a right for every American
- We cannot realize these principles without addressing the core problem of American health care: the systematic disengagement within our health care system of the economic tension that creates value. The path to genuine reform lies in finding workable and ethical ways to reestablish it.

- I'll attempt to develop logically how we can accomplish our goals in a way that's familiar and comfortable to Americans. We'll disengage American health care from employers and bureaucratic government programs and instead look to the highly successful model established by Social Security. We'll adapt and build on it, establishing:
  - A *standard* level of care that is a right for every American without regard to the ability to pay.
  - A *trust fund* dedicated to health care and funded with dedicated taxes for that purpose—a public financing of health care.
  - The design of *systems of care* which will become the basic building block of American health care—a completely private approach to its organization and delivery.
  - The *freedom* of every American to select the system of care they prefer, to pay for it with a voucher from the trust fund, and to extend their standard coverage with their own money if they choose.
  - Genuine *quality* by establishing robust medical practice standards and a continuous system of quality audits of the health care provided by each system of care.
  - This will create an adaptable, uniquely American health care system, with our economic system and creativity fully engaged to accomplish, not hinder, our goals of high quality and fair costs.

American health care, which has come so far in the last century, seems now to have lost its way. Its productivity has stagnated, with its growth in cost far outstripping its gain in effectiveness. Its blueprint is obsolete: a design for acute illness when chronic illness increasingly absorbs our resources and shortens our lives. Entrenched interests paralyze it just when it most needs to change and adapt. Its finances are unsustainable and threaten our nation's future. Like General Motors, its legacy of strength and great accomplishment has been eroded from within over the years by problems too quickly blamed on others or explained away rather than fixed. Also like GM, our nation has taken on large obligations without making provisions to pay for them. Unlike GM, however, there's nobody standing by to bail out America's health care system. We have to fix it ourselves.

I hoped that our new president would call us to the altar—would summon the almost infinite capacity of Americans, when they're asked, to do what needs to be done. It didn't happen. We have "reform" now but it didn't fix our problem. The new road we've chosen is far too much like the old one. When you've lost your way, you don't just speed up. You calm yourself, look around, and intelligently pick a direction.

There's still a great opportunity for American health care reform. We didn't follow most of our fellow industrial nations into a nationalized system after the Second World War. While some reformers look longingly at the lower costs and in some cases better results of those systems, that conservatism on our part might well prove to be a good thing. Here at the beginning of a new century we still have the possibility to learn from the experiences of others, to combine it with our own, to get our bearings, and fix the problem.

Why should I be writing this book? I'm not an academician, and even if I were inclined that way, I'm a sitting governor without the time to do the research that an academic treatment would demand. I have no desire to write an exposé or another recitation of problems in our health care system; this is well-plowed ground with many excellent works. Nor are my motives partisan: while I'm a Democrat, I'm not a particularly partisan one and have found solutions from a broad spectrum of ideological views over the years.

What I do have to offer though, is an unusual breadth and depth of direct experience with health care. Washington, probably inevitably, has become a land of secondhand knowledge. The "reform" we now have carries the strong imprint of that kind of knowledge: of national advocacy organizations, of well-educated and well-meaning legislative staffers, of the analysts of the Congressional Budget Office, of the ideologies of the union movement and the liberal wing of my own party. Each of these brings a valuable perspective. But as I watched the reform discussions unfold and took part in conversations with its designers, time and again I thought the conversations lacked the grounding and practicality that might have been provided by more *firsthand* knowledge. It's that perspective I can bring, and it leads me to different answers than those we've just found.

My views on health care—on what needs to be fixed and how we might accomplish that—have crystallized and evolved over the years, as I've engaged with the system on many fronts. As with most of us, some of that experience is personal. In the past five years, I've spent a night in an intensive care unit with what turned out to be a tick-borne disease, and got truly excellent medical care. I've also eulogized at the funerals of my younger and only brother and a brother-in-law, both of whom received some truly appalling primary care during their illnesses. My wife, Andrea, is a nurse and my daughter-in-law Dru, is a pediatric nurse practitioner. My half-brother, Dale, is a neurologist and runs a medical research institute on the West Coast.

I've been engaged for a long time with health care in the private sector. I've been a successful health care entrepreneur. In 1980, I started a company to manage health maintenance organizations on a table in my den and grew it to a public company with a million members and six thousand employees. I was the CEO of that company from its birth until it was sold. Along the way I spent a lot of evening hours working through issues with groups of doctors, negotiating with hospitals and labs and specialty groups, and discovering repeatedly and painfully all the various ways the medical industry has found to extract money from the health care system. This was my first brush with "reform": HMOs, if you will remember, were the great hope for health reform in the '70s and

'80s and I wanted to play. After the sale of my company, I took part in starting and managing other health care organizations. One of these was Coventry Corporation, where I was a founder and its first board chairman. Today it's a Fortune 500 managed care company with five million members. I took part in the start-up and management of other health care companies as well, including a dental HMO, a pharmacy benefits management company, and a specialized health information systems company.

I've been involved for many years in the public sector as well—in roles where I've had to balance budgets. As a governor, I had to take painful and controversial actions to keep TennCare—Tennessee's expansive Medicaid experiment in universal coverage—from bankrupting the state and saw firsthand how well-intentioned reforms can spin wildly out of control. To accomplish this, I had to negotiate with the federal government, fight over issues in the federal court system, reduce benefits, and, most painfully, remove people from health insurance coverage where the original reforms had overreached. I've learned a lot about both the strengths and limitations of advocacy groups. Following the TennCare reforms, I tried several new approaches to health insurance for the uninsured, including a small business product that's been successful and widely noted.

I've also taken part in national reform efforts. Governor Jim Douglas of Vermont and I have cochaired for several years the State Alliance for eHealth, and I've been an active member of the National Governors Association Executive Committee on these issues. The NGA Task Force on Health Reform represented the interests of the states in the evolution of the recent health reform, and I was one of the four governors—two Democrats and two Republicans—who spent many hours together on this subject. I've been the policy chair of the Democratic Governors Association for the past three years. While I have strong differences with my party on health reform, I'm not a political outlier—I've been a successful, moderately conservative, mainstream Democrat.

None of these experiences by itself is the window through which I look at health care. On the contrary, I believe the breadth and directness of my experience gives me a worthwhile and unusual perspective.

I do believe in the value of direct experience. To fix health care, at least some of the architects need to leave behind the policy conferences, roll up their sleeves, experience its messiness directly, and have some successes and—very important—some failures. The latter keeps your feet on the ground and the experience always improves the result.

This is a hard problem. If I were very overweight, settled into a comfortable and sedentary lifestyle, and my doctor were being honest with me, he'd sit me down and tell me that I really do have to shed some pounds and start moving around. My health and longevity depend on doing so. My honest doctor will also tell me that, much as I might wish to believe otherwise, there are no easy shortcuts. I have to change my lifestyle and that's hard.

Our health care system today is overweight and firmly settled in on a comfortable couch as well. Our nation's leadership needs to be just as honest and straightforward as that doctor, and tell us that health care really does have to shed some pounds and start moving about. The health of our nation depends on it. And those forthright political leaders would also tell us that, much as we'd like to believe otherwise, there are no easy shortcuts here either. Health care has to change its lifestyle and that's going to be hard.

An evolving America

Our American system of government is evolving into something not envisioned by our founders. It's not an exaggeration to say that the government we invented with our Constitution and refined over the years has now become, first of all, a vast social insurance system, with a side business in defense. I find this new role appropriate—a pragmatic and humane response to deep changes in our society. Others find it distasteful and I understand and respect that view. But whether or not you agree with this new role, it's a reality. Social Security and Medicare aren't going to go away. We've already crossed that bridge and engineered a deep change in the role of government. History will have to be the final judge of whether, in the end, we strengthened or diminished our people and our democracy.

We've accepted these new and different public sector responsibilities, but we haven't learned how to carry them out well. In the private sector, there's a Darwinian selection always at work. Everything is at risk and there are new ideas to challenge the old all the time. If things don't work or become obsolete, they tend to disappear. It happens very quickly in the world of the Internet and more slowly in enterprises such as the manufacture of automobiles. In the private sector, successful new ideas and products prosper and displace the old.

But the public sector is far less fluid. We've not changed with the times in the ways we manage our exploding health care responsibilities. Medicare and Medicaid were created in 1965 and reflected the views of the day as to how to finance and provide health care. Also in 1965, there were Rambler Americans on our roads everywhere. The Ramblers are long gone, and their replacements are very different and far more capable. However, the health reform we've just enacted looks very much like the Medicare and Medicaid programs of 1965. We've added millions of people to Medicaid, and subsidized millions of others to buy health insurance that looks a lot like Medicare. Neither program has shown any particular ability to deal with cost and quality issues over the years. In fact, the Congressional Budget Office has pointed out that during the period 1975–2005, the growth in adjusted per capita costs in both Medicare and Medicaid have exceeded those in other health sectors. Were this some private sector endeavor, we'd have long since begun moving on to something better designed and more efficient. In the public sector, however, we dutifully trot out these half-century-old ideas like one of those old Rambler Americans, fix a few dents, put on a coat of wax, and pronounce them once again our solution.

I'm approaching this problem with a straightforward logic: when it comes to health care, we've accepted broad government responsibility; our handling of that responsibility has been so weak as to put our nation deeply at risk; we need a new way to approach this. That different approach is very American: put our economic system to work to achieve our goals.

America has a long and distinguished history of innovation. But we in government need to remember just how creativity comes about. It requires stress, change, winners and losers, disruption, even a little anarchy. Government is necessarily almost the opposite. There's strong selection there for conformity and the very nature of government is to be a conservative force. We elect people to public office—myself included—who tend to play well with others (there are occasional exceptions!), and there's nothing about Washington (or Nashville, Albany, or Sacramento) that rewards disruption or even great creativity. Today's partisan shouting at one another across a chasm looks nothing like real creative tension or problem solving.

But if we're to assume these new and complex social responsibilities without bankrupting our nation, we need to engage that American talent for innovation. We need to allow for a touch of survival of the fittest—some winners and losers—as well. That's the problem I've set for myself in the pages ahead. I acknowledge we've accepted new responsibilities not foreseen by our founders. The old approach of elected officials, their staffs, and a coterie of lobbyists devising convoluted solutions isn't working—the scope and complexity is just too great.

We don't need our elected officials to design details; we need them to answer to a higher calling: leadership. We need them to show America the need to face up to the realities of our health care system and the financial dangers it presents to us. When they've done so, we also need an answer about where we go from here. My offering to our leadership in this book is this: that the answer lies in subtlety. Don't try to solve the problem yourself. Move up a level and figure out, instead, how to create the conditions—the stress, the fluidity, the incentives, the Darwinian tension—in which America's muscular economic system and the vast creative forces that inhabit our land are put back to work.

I

A Contrarian View

. . . in which we express our disappointment.

January 20, 2009

It was my second presidential inauguration; my first was Bill Clinton's in 1993.

Back then, I was in the crowd a couple hundred yards from the tiny figures on the Capitol steps. This time, as a sitting governor, the experience was very different. I was seated right there, on the podium, looking out over the crowd of a million people.

As noon approached, it was still cold, and as I looked down the Mall over the crowd there was dust and a little smoke in the air that made it shimmering and golden in the distance. I'd expected an experience that was completely in the moment; the sense of being present *now*, at a very particular milestone of history, recorded in a thousand ways, with recognizable figures of the day everywhere.

Instead, it was just the opposite, and in the middle of all the energy there was a silence and a mystical sense of timelessness and possibility. I believe that Providence favors America, and that when we need guidance there's a door that opens for a moment to give us a fresh glimpse of what we might aspire to. Sitting on that stage, feeling that timelessness, I imagined that if I shut my eyes a moment I might open them to that same yellow sunlight, but the year would be 1861. Civil War would be upon us, we'd be waiting for Abraham Lincoln, and if we listened carefully we might be able to hear that door open. Or it could be 1933, our economic system in shambles, and we'd be waiting for Franklin D. Roosevelt.

I had supported, campaigned, and voted for the man about to become our president, but had sometimes been publicly critical as well. I both admired and had reservations about Barack Obama. I admired his personal story and his extraordinary ability to inspire. I had reservations about what seemed to me an elitist view of the world and his brief political experience. But now, sitting there, awaiting the noon hour, the reservations melted away and I *believed*. A new kind of president, gifted with intelligence and eloquence, was taking the helm of a deeply challenged nation, one hungry for change. It was a transcendental moment. I believed, and as I sat there I thought I could hear that door opening once again.

Back in the present, on the inaugural stage the new president was sworn in, we all shook hands, traded a story or two, and went off to watch the parade. I thought, like a lot of Americans, that the time had arrived when our nation would confront some deep problems, high among them a health care system that was bankrupting our nation. Good omens are everywhere: in a terrible economy, business leaders who had opposed reform in the past are now feeling the full effect of health care costs to their competitiveness and financial well-being. Many Americans live in families facing layoffs and for the first time are staring in the face the very real possibility of being without. A growing number of people from all walks of life and ideologies are alarmed about our enormous deficit. They know that the problem is complex, but also that it can't be solved without addressing health care.

And now, at just this time, we have a new president who has made solving this problem his first domestic priority. He brings a powerful mandate to strike out in fresh directions. He clearly aspires to be a transformational leader. The American people are ready. The mood in the country reminds me of the mood in the weeks following the attacks of September 11: *tell us what to do.*

Fourteen months later: March 23, 2010

What a stunning disappointment.

The health care "reform" we finally wrote into law isn't transformational. It provides health insurance for a great many more people, but doesn't directly attack any of the deep structural problems of health care. There's a lot of tinkering, but the tough problems—cost, sustainability, inconsistent quality, fragmentation, the focus on heroic interventions—remain placidly untransformed. It's as if we had inherited a proud old house that had deteriorated over the years. Now it's in disrepair—sagging floors, rusty pipes, and costing a fortune to maintain. But rather than rolling up our sleeves and strengthening the beams and joists, we choose to tack a cobbled-together addition on the back, slap a coat of paint on everything, and pronounce it fixed.

Our "reform" wasn't transformational, nor was it especially courageous. The planets were aligned: for a moment, Americans were attentive, were ready to listen and to try new things. We were ready for change. But neither the president nor Congress—and I include both parties here—were willing to talk plainly and honestly to the American people. They were unwilling to tell us things we didn't want to hear or to call on us to do anything hard. Instead, with a great deal of drama, they added some new taxes, but only on the rich, and did some creative bookkeeping. This let them make the claim that this, too, was really pretty much free. With that out of the way, they added tens of millions more people—deserving people—into a broken and unsustainable system, and asked for applause.

I've learned to practice the political arts over the years and believe I understand fully that politics, at its heart, is the "art of the possible." Even seen through that practical filter, what we finally accomplished is still a deep disappointment. We had a new president with honorable intentions, vision, a clear desire to fix the system and the world's best political brand to bring to bear. Instead—for reasons that seem almost inexplicable to me—he turned the problem over to Congress. I've come to respect very much the role that legislatures play in our system of government. But I've also learned that, even if they're filled with brilliant and constructive members, there are some things they just can't do. One of those things is to invent coherent and focused solutions to complicated problems. Structurally, it doesn't work: there are just too many people with too many diverse ideas. It's like trying to write a good novel with dozens of authors who all have different ideas of what the novel is about. Legislatures are valuable, but they're better editors than authors.

Congress accepted the problem, and tried to solve it with the script they reliably use: redefine the problem in ideological terms, avoid any hard decisions that aren't immediately necessary, appropriate money, protect friends, and punish enemies. The end product was technically competent and did some good things, but managed to sidestep most of the genuinely difficult issues that sooner or later we have to confront. Surely in America, the most innovative country in the world, we can do better with such an opportunity. Perhaps I'd been wrong that winter day in front of the Capitol. Perhaps that door and its fresh glimpse of what America might aspire to didn't appear this time. Or perhaps it did, for a moment, but our attention was too consumed with the trivia of politics to look up and accept the gift.

The Patient Protection and Affordable Care Act of 2010

The Patient Protection and Affordable Care Act is a lengthy and complex piece of legislation with a convoluted history. Because of its complexity and the partisan nature of so much of the commentary on it, it's easy to become confused with just what it does and how it's paid for. Before I explain why I believe it to be inadequate, let me begin by attempting to organize and summarize what the legislation does and how it's paid for in as neutral a fashion as I can.

The final shape of the president's health reform is the result of two pieces of legislation. In December 2009, the Senate had passed its version of health reform legislation on a narrow party-line vote (60–39). That legislation, however, was unacceptable to a large number of House Democrats. But with the election the following month of Republican Scott Brown in Massachusetts, the Democrats no longer had the sixty votes necessary to pass new health reform legislation in the Senate. The compromise between Senate and House Democrats was to have the House pass the Senate version, but with an understanding of changes that would be made through the "reconciliation" process. This is a parliamentary process that would modify the original legislation without needing sixty votes in the Senate. The Senate reform bill that was approved by the House was the "Patient Protection and Affordable Care Act of 2010"; the companion legislation was the "Health Care and Education Reconciliation Act of 2010." The former was signed into law by the president on March 23, 2010, the latter on March 30. For convenience, I'm going to refer to these two pieces of legislation taken together from now on as the "Affordable Care Act." This is President Obama's health care reform.

If we step back and simplify—look for the big shapes—there are three of them, and the rest I would characterize more or less as miscellany. Those three big shapes that define the framework of what the Affordable Care Act does are:

- It creates a mandate, requiring as a matter of law that nearly every American have an approved level of health insurance or pay a penalty.
- It establishes a system of federal subsidies to completely or partially pay for the now required health insurance for about thirty-four million Americans who are currently uninsured.

These subsidies are made available through a combination of expanding the existing Medicaid program and creating new entities called *Exchanges*. In addition, several million Americans who currently have health insurance are expected to convert to subsidized coverage through the Exchanges.

• It places extensive new requirements on the health insurance industry.

Mandate. The first big shape is the creation of a so-called "mandate"—a legal requirement that nearly every American citizen and legal resident must have health insurance or pay a penalty. This is a feature of the Affordable Care Act that has provoked considerable opposition from those who believe it represents an overreaching of federal power. The legislation also defines in broad terms, with details to be filled in by the secretary of Health and Human Services, minimum requirements for what an individual's health insurance has to cover in order for that individual to legally meet the mandate requirements. Those minimum requirements look much like one of today's moderately broad conventional health insurance policies, with a notable additional emphasis on access to preventive care.

There are financial penalties in the form of a new tax on individuals who fail to buy health insurance and a penalty on employers above a certain size who don't cover their employees. The Internal Revenue Service is the agency charged with enforcement. Those penalties on individuals, after a brief start-up period, are $695 annually for each individual (limited to three times that amount for any family) or 2.5% of income, whichever is greater. An individual without the required insurance and with an income of $20,000 pays a tax of $695; at $50,000 the tax is $1,250; at $100,000 it's $2,500. There are a number of exceptions to the requirement to buy health insurance, including various forms of financial hardship, being without coverage for three months or less, being an American Indian, or being in prison.

Subsidies. The second large shape in the Affordable Care Act—and where most of the money goes—is a system of subsidies for the purchase of health insurance that are based primarily on income and family size. The mandate will inevitably create a large group of Americans who are obligated to buy health insurance but who can't afford it. These subsidies are designed to assist them in meeting their obligation, and they fall into three categories.

The first subsidy is a complete one—an expansion of the existing Medicaid program to include every American whose income is under "133% of poverty." Each year the Department of Health and Human Services (HHS) defines and publishes guidelines establishing a level of annual income below which a family in America is considered to be living in poverty. This number depends on the size of the family and in 2010, for example, it is $10,830 for a single individual and $22,050 for a family of four. The "133% of poverty" jargon simply describes an income equal to 1.33 times the poverty level guideline that's in effect (in the Affordable Care Act it's actually 1.38 times the poverty guideline due to a separate additional provision in the law). What this means in practical terms is that when this Medicaid expansion takes place, beginning in 2014, individuals with incomes less than about $15,800 or families of four with incomes less than about $32,300 will become eligible for comprehensive and nearly free health insurance.

Prior to the implementation of the Affordable Care Act, in order to be eligible for Medicaid a citizen had to meet three tests. First, there was an income test: an individual had to have (or be part of a family that had) an income below certain levels. Individual states exercise considerable discretion today as to what those income levels are and therefore who is covered. Some states have used Medicaid broadly, with generous income limits, while others have taken much more limited approaches. Second, an individual had to meet an asset test. While it varies by state, to be eligible for Medicaid an individual's assets had to be less than a few thousand dollars. Those who had low income but still owned assets above the limit had to first spend those assets to qualify. (This is an issue primarily with long-term care, where there's a considerable industry in finding ways to use Medicaid to pay for nursing home care while preserving an elderly person's assets—typically a house—for heirs.) Third, an individual had to be a member of one of the covered *categories* of individuals: children, pregnant women, or a person who is disabled, for example.

The Affordable Care Act changes all this. There will now be a national uniform income qualification—having an income below the "133% of poverty" level—and there's no longer any requirement to spend other assets or to belong to a covered category. The primary effect on Medicaid of the new law will be to make eligible large numbers of lower income adults who had previously been excluded by law. It also opens eligibility to those whose income is temporarily low but have assets, for example, families with a home and automobile where the breadwinner has been laid off. The philosophical change is substantial: Medicaid has always in effect made a distinction between the "deserving poor" (for example, the aged, blind, disabled, children, some single parents, pregnant women) and the "undeserving poor" (able-bodied adults). This distinction, which some consider a Victorian-era holdover and others consider quintessentially American, is now gone. The Affordable Care Act expansion of Medicaid eligibility is expected to provide health insurance to approximately eighteen million additional Americans by 2019.

The second of these subsidies, and the most discussed, is an extensive cost-sharing arrangement for health insurance purchased through new "Exchanges." The Exchanges are designed to be state-run administrative organizations that will organize and approve health insurance plans being sold by the insurance industry and present those plans accurately and in one place as a form of "one-stop shopping." Their goal is transparency—presenting consumers with accurate information to allow them to easily understand and compare plans. This is expected to foster competition among insurers for a consumer's business. The health insurance offered through these Exchanges is primarily available to those without employer-provided health insurance. I'd hazard a guess that these Exchanges and the related system of subsidies will be seen a decade from now as overwhelmingly the dominant and most important feature of the Affordable Care Act.

While consumers legally have to buy insurance that covers all the required services, they'll have the flexibility to choose among plans that cover different fractions of the total cost of those services. The Affordable Care Act defines four tiers of insurance based on the percentage of a person's health care costs that are expected to be covered by the insurance itself: these levels are called in the legislation "bronze" (60% of the expected health care costs covered by the insurance), "silver" (70%), "gold" (80%), and "platinum" (90%). The "silver" plan is used as the reference plan in calculating how much subsidy is available to a purchaser.

The Exchanges will undoubtedly facilitate comparison shopping. Their major impact, however, will be that a great many of the insurance policies bought through the Exchange will benefit from substantial federal subsidies. These subsidies are available to Americans whose income is up to "400% of poverty" ($93,700 for a family of four in 2014). They're designed to limit the health care expenses for an individual buying a "silver" plan on a sliding percentage scale. At "133% of poverty," an individual is responsible for the cost of health insurance up to a level of 2% of their income. For incomes above this level, the maximum percentage of income that anyone should have to pay increases in steps to 9.5% of income at "400% of poverty." Table 1 provides some examples of how the cost of health insurance purchased through the Exchange would be divided between the consumer and the federal subsidy.

In addition, there are provisions in the Affordable Care Act limiting the amount of out-of-pocket expenses that a family will have to bear. This second form of subsidy provides substantial additional

Table 1
Exchange Cost Sharing 2014

Family Income		Cost of Insurance		
Amount	Percentage of Poverty	Individual Cost	Federal Subsidy	Subsidy Percent of Total
$ 30,000	128	0	$ 19,300*	100
40,000	171	$ 1,982	12,263	86
50,000	213	3,385	10,860	76
60,000	256	4,937	9,308	65
70,000	299	6,626	7,619	53
80,000	342	7,600	6,645	47
90,000	384	8,550	5,695	40
100,000	427	14,245	0	0

Source: Kaiser Family Foundation "Health Reform Subsidy Calculator"
http://healthreform.kff.org/SubsidyCalculator.aspx

Note: Based on purchase of the "silver" plan (70% actuarial value), family of four, forty-five-year-old policyholder, medium cost area, health insurance policy cost of $14,245 (estimated by Kaiser) in 2014.

*A family with $30,000 of income would qualify for Medicaid, which is not directly comparable to the Exchange Policies. It would not typically have premium costs and out-of-pocket costs vary by state. This figure is an estimate based on Medicaid having a value of 95% of the total cost of health care.

value to families in the lower and middle regions of the income scale. For a family with an income of about $40,000 in 2014, these provisions increase the actuarial value of a typical silver health insurance plan by roughly another $2,500 in addition to the $12,000 premium subsidy. In other words, a family of four with an income of around $40,000 that purchases insurance through the Exchange will be subsidized in total about $14,500. These Exchanges are expected to enroll about twenty-nine million Americans by 2019, with about ten million of those being conversions from existing insurance coverage.

Finally, the third subsidy consists of temporary (two-year) tax credits to small businesses as an incentive to begin offering health insurance. The credit can be up to 50% of the employer's contribution in businesses with fewer than ten employees and an average wage under $25,000. The credit declines with larger size and higher wages until it disappears at twenty-five employees or a $50,000 annual income average. I should also note that while there's no legal mandate for employers to offer insurance, there are penalties for employers of over fifty persons who don't offer insurance or whose insurance places too much of the cost on the employee. Depending on the exact circumstances, these penalties are in $2,000–$3,000 per employee range. These anticipated penalties are a substantial source of the revenue that is used to pay for the Affordable Care Act.

New insurance industry requirements. The third large shape in the Affordable Care Act is a set of new insurance industry requirements that substantially alter the business model of the industry. Many of these changes would be broadly accepted as desirable and with the Affordable Care Act become practical. The Affordable Care Act requires insurers to issue policies to anyone qualified who applies, to renew policies without regard to the health status of the insured, to eliminate pre-existing condition limitations, and to require that rates in the Exchange and small group markets vary only based on age, the geographic area, family composition, and tobacco use. The broader insurance coverage made possible by the Affordable Care Act considerably reduces the adverse selection problems that made these changes impractical before. ("Adverse selection" is the insurance term corresponding to the common-sense observation that the business of providing home-owner insurance for someone's house doesn't work if the home owner gets to call up and buy it at standard rates when the hurricane is on the way.)

There are other requirements on the insurance industry that are more arbitrary in nature and reflect, in part, the political dynamic of the industry having been made the enemy in health reform. For example, insurance companies will have to pay providers at least 85% of the premiums they collect from large groups for medical care and there are new review processes for rate increases deemed "excessive."

The actuary at the federal Centers for Medicare and Medicaid Services estimates that the combined effects of the mandate, subsidies, and changes in the insurance industry will make available health insurance for up to thrity-four million more Americans and thereby reduce the number of uninsured to about twenty-three million by 2019.

The Affordable Care Act also contains dozens of provisions in addition to those related directly to covering the uninsured. A few of them are substantial: improvements in the Medicare Part D benefit (the Medicare pharmacy program) at a ten-year cost of $40 billion and increasing payment rates to primary care providers at a cost of $8.3 billion, for example. A great many are modest (at least in federal terms): the Money Follows the Person Federal Rebalancing Demonstration Program at a cost of $1.7 billion is a typical example. There are also a large number of more minor provisions: a small sampling would include Medicare coverage for individuals exposed to environmental hazards ($300 million), data collection on health disparities ($200 million), improvements to the physician feedback program ($100 million), and the Elder Justice Coordinating Council ($28 million). Taken together, these additional items are considerable but neither these costs nor some additional projected savings are generally considered in the calculation of the Affordable Care Act's effect on the deficit.

Politically, and to conform to the president's stated objective, health reform had to show that it wouldn't "increase the deficit." As Congress considered the legislation in the spring of 2010, the Congressional Budget Office (CBO) issued a report on March 20 stating that the proposed expansion of coverage and its offsetting taxes and savings would produce a net reduction in the deficit over the next ten years (the CBO's mandated time horizon) of $124 billion. That deficit reduction number was modified by a subsequent CBO letter on May 11 that estimated the Affordable Care Act would require about an additional $115 billion to fund items not originally scored. At that time there still remained a further fifty-three line items that were also authorized but not yet scored.

The financial effects of this legislation are complex under any circumstances, and have been made more so by the practice of focusing on the single measurement of the Affordable Care Act's net effect on the deficit rather than the actual costs, savings, and new revenues that it's expected

Table 2
Ten-Year Financial Summary
Uninsured Coverage Expansion Provisions of the Affordable Care Act

Source of Funds	$ billions
Taxes and fines	$ 517
Reduced payments to providers	368
Use of initial CLASS premiums	70
Other revenue and savings	133
Total Source of Funds	$ 1,088
New Expenditures	
Medicaid expansion (with CHIP)	$ 434
Exchange subsidies	465
Small-employer tax credits	37
Overhead and other	47
Total New Expenditures	$ 983
Expansion-related "deficit reduction"	$ 105

Sources: Elmsdorf to Pelosi, March 20, 2010,
http://www.cbo.gov/ftpdocs/113xx/doc11379/AmendReconProp.pdf;
Elmsdorf to Lewis, May 11, 2010,
http://www.cbo.gov/ftpdocs/114xx/doc11490/LewisLtr_HR3590.pdf; Joint Committee on Taxation, *Estimated Revenue Effects of the Amendment..etc., Document JCX-17-10, http://www.jct.gov/publications.html?func=download&id=3672&chk=bed1ec995cob2d 1c815c60do516bade7&no_html=1*

Notes: This table addresses the "coverage expansion" costs of the Affordable Care Act as defined by the Congressional Budget office (CBO), and adds an additional $17 million to the expenditures to reflect the additional administrative costs clearly associated with the coverage expansion, as stated by the CBO on May 11, 2010. It respects the CBO conventions as to what items from the legislation are to be scored for the purpose of deficit analysis; the numbers in this table are those provided by the CBO without editorial adjustment.

to produce. Table 2 summarizes the costs, and the means of paying them, of the Affordable Care Act's expansion of insurance coverage.

Supporters of the Affordable Care Act take considerable pride in the fact that it will make health insurance available to another thirty-four million Americans, and they should. I'll step out of my temporarily neutral role now, and applaud that. That's a lot of citizens who won't have to go to emergency rooms or charitable clinics every time they need medical attention, who'll get preventive care, who'll have continuity in their medical care, and who won't be forced into bankruptcy by unexpected health problems.

This isn't a policy issue for me; it's a very personal one. My only full sibling, my younger brother, Dean, died several years ago, in his late fifties. For most of his life he didn't have health insurance or a personal physician and he died from diseases arising from personal choices: heavy smoking and alcohol abuse. I don't know for sure that having better access to health care would have saved him, but I can imagine a lot of ways in which it might have. I would have liked for him to have had that chance. It is no small thing to have invited Dean and tens of millions of other Americans into our health care system. It should have been done decades ago and I'm proud that we've now taken a large step toward accomplishing it.

The problem isn't that we expanded coverage. The problem is that expanding coverage is about all we did.

2

What's Wrong with Reform

. . . in which we consider why the Patient Protection and Affordable Care Act of 2010 fails to meet our nation's needs.

Health care issues have become very difficult. I begin with a great deal of respect for anyone who tries to address them, whether it was former Governor Romney in Massachusetts or is President Obama in Washington. But trying and doing are not the same thing, and so far we've fallen well short of giving our nation what it needs.

This is a contrarian view for a Democrat, and I need to justify it. Many of my fellow elected officials, including some whose understanding of health care I respect very much, believe strongly that our nation, and Democrats in particular, have achieved an historic success. They believe that the years ahead will vindicate the direction taken, and that this reform has set in motion forces that will solve our health care problems. Before we move on to the real focus of this book, I want to spend some time laying out my reasons for this dissenting view.

My disappointment with the Affordable Care Act can be summarized in nine words: *when conditions are good you do the hard things.* The conditions were certainly good—with a new, intelligent, persuasive president and a public eager for fresh directions—for change. But we didn't do the hard things. Expanding coverage is important, but we also face very large and difficult problems with the cost of health care. If we're to get anywhere close to financial sustainability in our health care system—which we have to do sooner rather than later—there are major and difficult steps we need to take to control costs and to actually pay for what we are using now. We didn't do that, and there are plenty of ways in which we made things worse. I wish there was a Will Rogers around Washington today. Here's what he said before the stock market crash of 1929:

"You will try to show us that we are prosperous, because we have more. I will show you where we are not prosperous, because we haven't paid for it yet."

I have other concerns as well: we passed on the chance to simplify and strengthen our health care system and instead added new layers of bureaucracy and complexity. As a public official who believes in being frank with the public, it bothers me that we presented the costs of reform to the public in a too-clever way. We had a chance to use this issue to bridge some partisan divides, but instead we burned some of the few bridges we already had.

Paying for health care

We *have* to fix the finances of our health care system—both public and private. America is on a dangerous collision course with fiscal reality that we can't ignore much longer. To remind us: in 2008 our Medicare program alone had unfunded liabilities of around $37 trillion. That means that we've legally promised to pay for $37 trillion (in today's dollars) more in health care costs—just for our elderly—than we have funds provided through our taxes to pay for. To put that in perspective, that represents a current obligation of about $280,000 for every full-time worker in America. No one has any taste for imposing the kinds of tax increases that it would take to pay for this—and even if we did, it would be a crushing blow to our economy. There's a limit, even for America, as to how much we can borrow. To make matters worse, the trends are awful; that unfunded Medicare liability has almost tripled in just the last eight years.

We give this problem lip service, but we don't do anything about it. Over the years, I've been to a great many conferences and panels to discuss health care issues. They follow a stylized pattern. There's an obligatory sequence at the opening that acknowledges our tremendous cost problem and shows a chart or two. It's almost a required element, like the opening action sequence in a James Bond film. Then, having uttered the obligatory words, the discussion rapidly proceeds to other matters such as who's going to pay to add more people and benefits.

It's not just a federal issue. The states have a share of this problem in the form of Medicaid—health care for lower income Americans—which is a joint responsibility of the federal government and the several states. Many of us in state government are already finding our commitments to be very difficult to maintain. States are being put in a box. Most are prohibited from borrowing money to balance budgets and Medicaid increasingly shoulders aside investments in other areas such as education and infrastructure. In Tennessee, Medicaid didn't exist in 1965, in 1981 its budget was about half of what we spent on K–12 education, it surpassed spending on K–12 in 1992, and by 2004 it was 2.25 times our K–12 budget. With the Affordable Care Act, it will get worse.

A lost opportunity to control costs

This year's reform presented a fine opportunity to make some progress in containing the costs of our health care and we passed it up. The Affordable Care Act is primarily about expanding the number of people covered and establishing federal subsidies. Its attention to controlling costs is limited, in the future, and has an air of wishful thinking about it. It contains a host of grants to "pilot" various ideas, it encourages the creation of "accountable care" organizations and it subsidizes information technology. The cost-reducing element that is most highlighted is the creation of an Independent Payment Advisory Board (IPAB). This board is charged with making recommendations for holding down Medicare spending any time it grows at a rate of more than 1% over general inflation. We already have a similar board, the Medical Payment Advisory Commission (Med-PAC), which has been doing this for some time—it was established by the Balanced Budget Act of 1997. The difference between Med-PAC and IPAB is that the IPAB recommendations will automatically go into effect unless Congress makes offsetting cuts or has sixty votes to override the recommendations. President Obama has called it "MedPAC on steroids."

But it would be prudent to be skeptical that any recommendation with enough bite to really make a difference will actually be implemented. Exhibit A is what has happened with a single previous reduction: in this case Medicare physician payment rates. Since 2002, Congress has continuously overridden a reduction that it had previously made in those rates—this is the so-called annual "doc fix"—and has found no difficulty in finding the required votes to do so whether Republicans or Democrats were running the show. As I'm finalizing this manuscript, Congress has just extended the "doc fix" again for another six months.

Even if I'm wrong, even if all these longer-term techniques work, we're still a long way from addressing the cost problem. We talk about "not increasing the deficit," which is Washington speak. The structural deficit is expanding and will continue to expand at a dangerous rate. All that phrase means is the questionable claim that the Affordable Care Act won't make it any worse. Former Office of Management and Budget Director Peter Orszag, who is a strong supporter of the Affordable Care Act, and for whom I have great respect, believes that it will hold the proportion of GDP devoted to health care ½% below what it would have been without the Act. Even if he's correct, that means that while health care costs were projected to become 25% of our economy in the 20s, it might only be 24.5%. Neither comes close to working.

When the Affordable Care Act was being considered, there were plenty of cost containment strategies that were ready to go and didn't require pilot projects or new commissions. One obvious example is the federal government's prohibiting its own Medicare and Medicaid agencies from negotiating prices with pharmaceutical companies. The Affordable Care Act could have reversed that and begun treating the purchase of pharmaceuticals like the purchase of everything else, saving billions of dollars annually in the process. The reason that drugs are less expensive in Canada isn't a secret: their government negotiates prices.

MedPac reports to Congress regularly, and those reports contain dozens of realistic and effective cost-containment strategies that could have been incorporated and produced immediate, not long-term, savings. As an example, in their June 2010 report, MedPac discussed pharmaceutical products that treat osteoarthritis:

"The Congressional Budget Office (CBO) included as a policy option use of the least costly alternative approach to pay for five products that physicians use to treat osteoarthritis of the knee. Although each product differs slightly, they are all approved by the Food and Drug Administration for the same indication—osteoarthritis—and they work through the same clinical mechanism. CBO estimated savings of about $200 million between 2010 and 2014 and almost $500 million between 2010 and 2019 if Medicare set the payment for these five products based on the lowest priced product" (Congressional Budget Office 2008).

The concept of paying only the cost of the least expensive drug in any group of equivalent drugs is called "reference pricing." It could have been enforced for this, and many other groups of drugs, with a line or two in the legislation.

I should note that this specific recommendation actually stopped well short of everything that could be done in this single area to reduce costs without affecting patient care. Paying for every drug at the price of the least expensive is an improvement, but doesn't really give a pharmaceutical company much incentive to keep prices down. They get the same amount of business and profit wherever they set their price. If Medicare were to take the next step, however, and pay *only* for the drug that was the lowest price, there would be a strong incentive on pharmaceutical companies to lower prices. The lowest price would get five times the business. When I was trying to solve our problems with the TennCare program in Tennessee in 2005, I proposed exactly this to the federal government for a few groups of drugs and got nowhere; this was in what was supposed to be a conservative administration.

This entire issue of being selective about paying for higher priced treatments when there's no evidence that they are any better is a rich field for holding down costs. That same MedPAC report discussed two different treatments for certain kinds of cancer with no evidence of any difference in their success; one is $20,000, the other $40,000. In most areas of economic life, whether public or private, if there are two equivalent products and one is much more expensive than the other, you have a lot of explaining and justifying to do if you buy the more expensive. In health care, it's just the opposite: you have to explain and justify in order to limit the purchase to the less expensive alternative.

The point here is that there's already an abundance of good ways to reduce medical expenses, right now, with no harmful effects on care. But the real ones make someone mad: one person's excess cost is someone else's livelihood. So we leave alone the ways that fight back and go after "administrative costs," or "giving doctors better information," or starting pilot projects. In a competitive economy like ours, it surprises me that so many otherwise sensible people place an easy faith in the success of some of these soft, cooperative approaches. There's a fundamental economic reality here: no one—doctors, hospitals, pharmaceutical companies, or anyone else—is going to work cooperatively with us to reduce their income. That's a naive view: life doesn't work that way.

Until we accept that solving the health care cost problem is going to create conflict, make various interests mad, and result in winners and losers, we won't get anywhere. I'll argue in a later chapter that government is probably incapable of doing this, and propose another way. But if government *can* do it—if it can be tough enough to genuinely begin to reduce costs—we just had the best shot to do so in many years and missed.

Adding to the cost of health care

We failed to use the opportunity to address the cost issue substantively. Worse yet, we also did some things likely to make our health care obligations even more expensive in the years ahead.

First, for anyone qualifying for a federal subsidy, the financial terms of health insurance purchased through an Exchange are extremely attractive. A consequence of that is, it seems likely to me, that Exchanges will attract many more buyers of its subsidized insurance than expected. As you'll remember, for most people an Exchange provides subsidies up to "400% of poverty." That income qualification encompasses a very large number of people, over 60% of America's under-sixty-five population and over 80% of the uninsured population. Most of those who are now uninsured (and choose to buy insurance rather than pay a penalty) will use the Exchange. Many people who are already purchasing insurance in the individual market will do so as well. Both of those effects are anticipated in the cost calculations provided by the CBO.

But subsidized Exchange health insurance is structured to be so much more attractive than other alternatives that I believe it's likely to grow, and with it the federal entitlement subsidies, far beyond the scope that was originally anticipated. What will make it grow is a third group that can potentially enter—those who now have group insurance.

There are a lot of businesses—small, medium, and large—in America that, when they do the numbers, are going to discover that dropping the health insurance coverage they now offer and moving their employees into the Individual Exchange program is better for them and better for their employees. They'll no longer feel a moral obligation to maintain coverage, as there are no longer restrictions that would prevent any of their employees from smoothly moving to new coverage. For lower-wage (and plenty of medium-wage) employees, that employee's share of the cost of coverage through the Exchange will be less than their contribution to the employer plan. The employee's paycheck goes *up* if she can move. For a great many employers, when they compare the total costs of dropping coverage with those of keeping it, dropping it will make good financial sense. Even today, there's already significant erosion of group health insurance as firms face economic pressure. Once there's a clear path that doesn't hurt their employees; dropping coverage will be a very attractive option. Furthermore, there are many employers (including many state and local governments) who have substantial costs associated with health coverage for retirees who have not yet reached sixty-five. By definition, these are expensive individuals as they're at the older end of the age spectrum. Where these benefits are not being paid as a contractual obligation, moving these retired employees to the Exchanges will be an attractive alternative. In Tennessee, where we pay these costs but have no contractual obligation to do so, our expected costs are about $1.7 billion and some future governor could use the Exchange to quickly eliminate a good deal of that liability (and its increases in the future). I'm confident that many employers are looking hard at these options now, and by 2014 there will be a mini-industry of consultants to show them how to do it and what they can save.

The strategy for start-up and very small companies seems even clearer. If someone were starting a company in 2014, it would be a perfectly sensible business decision for them to decide right at the start to permanently stay out of the business of offering health insurance. A company with one or two dozen employees—and there are a lot of those—might do so as well. They're not taking anything away, they just tell their employees that health insurance is their responsibility and introduce them to the Exchange. Perhaps they'll enhance their employee's paychecks a little to cover their portion of the cost. As these small businesses grow, some will reach a size where fines would start to apply, but a fine of two or three thousand dollars will look very attractive as an alternative to a contribution of $15,000 or more for an employer-sponsored family policy. For top executives, the business can always provide extra benefits or wrap-around coverage with after-tax dollars. The limited and brief tax credits provided for in the Affordable Care Act are no competition for this strategy. While Congress might eventually attempt to short-circuit this approach by raising the fines, most businesses would sensibly decide to take their chances, confident that the politics of such a move and the clout of business lobbyists in Washington would still protect them.

This isn't going to be a small effect. Employers with tens of millions of employees in their organizations are going to take a hard look at this. It represents a genuine design flaw in the Exchange system—setting up the economic incentives to favor exactly what you don't want: employers dumping into the federal system. Perhaps it's an oversight by the designers who aren't really attached to the world where nickels and dimes count. Or it may be just what they're counting on, as a back-door approach to a government-run system.

Let me make a prediction here: *subsidized, Individual Exchange–based health insurance is an open-ended entitlement that will ultimately, and perhaps quite quickly, create extremely large and unbudgeted costs for our federal government.*

The second area where the Affordable Care Act is likely to increase health costs is more subtle. Forcing more competition on the health insurance industry through Exchanges sounds good in the abstract—what could be wrong with additional competition? But there are two sides to health care transactions. As the dominance of a few large insurers in a market diminishes, more economic power accrues to providers, and especially large providers. Their ability to dictate rates and terms grows. Forcing competition and fragmentation among those paying for care while simultaneously encouraging cooperation and consolidation among providers will cause medical costs to go up, not down. Moreover, new constraints placed on the insurance industry in the name of reform hinder the insurers' ability and incentive to innovate.

The power to determine rates that providers with a dominant position in a market enjoy is very real. Massachusetts Attorney General Martha Coakley issued a preliminary report on these anti-competitive effects in early 2010. It found that price variations were not correlated with quality, sickness, the mix of Medicare or Medicaid patients, or whether the facility was a teaching facility or not. What the price variations *did* correlate with was the market leverage of the institution relative to other providers.

Similarly, in California, Robert Berenson, Paul Ginsburg, and Nicole Kemper wrote, in *Health Affairs,* in the spring of 2010 about the same difficulties with market concentration in California. They described the phenomenon of "must have" hospitals: ones that must be included in the network to make it acceptable to consumers. Their poster child is Cedars-Sinai Medical Center in Los Angeles, a "must-have" hospital with the "highest rates in the world." They describe group practice fee increases in the double digits annually and quoted one physician in a powerful group lamenting facetiously that "the last annual rate increases for his group had 'deteriorated' from 20% to 'only' 12%." This "must have" provider effect is particularly strong with children's hospitals and subspecialty groups where there may be only one in the service area.

These findings in Massachusetts and California are not news to anyone who has ever negotiated rates with the provider community. The Affordable Care Act pushes the consolidation of hospitals and provider groups while disarming the purchasers. As this market power disparity between purchasers and providers grows, we can expect medical costs in many markets to go up at rates in excess of even the already high rate of health care inflation. This won't be due to health care's usual suspects of technology or overutilization, but just because of good old-fashioned monopoly market power.

The third area in which the Affordable Care Act is likely to increase costs is the portion of the act that creates the CLASS Act (that's the Community Living Assistance Services and Supports program). This less-noticed aspect of the legislation is something that Senator Ted Kennedy had sought for a long time. It creates an entirely new entitlement apart from the coverage expansion for the uninsured. It's a voluntary, nationwide insurance program, paid for through payroll deductions, to help provide assistance to the elderly who need long-term services and support. This is a very good idea if it's honestly financed. It was presented in the reform legislation as a self-financing program, with the insurance premiums fully paying for the benefits. But its terms quite obviously open it to strong adverse selection—signing up a disproportionate number of sick people. The ink was hardly dry on the Affordable Care Act before the CMS actuary stated that the CLASS Act would be out of money by about 2025. At that point, we will have been taking our citizens' good faith premium payments for ten years. We're not going to fail to honor our obligations and we can expect to be subsidizing this entitlement in growing amounts in the years ahead.

Even associates of mine who strongly support the Affordable Care Act acknowledge privately that its main purpose has been expanding coverage. Their argument is that we need to do the expansions now and we'll revisit costs once the new coverage is in place. But this is a terrible strategy. When a business executive needs something from her union (or vice versa) the time to ask is when she has something to give. We've just added a trillion dollars into our health care system that, among other things, eliminates a good deal of the need for physicians and hospitals to provide care to the uninsured without compensation. As a minimum, we should have demanded and gotten in return some movement on pricing and utilization.

I don't know when the next opportunity will arise to do some of the tough things required with health care costs. I acknowledge that there are some small and tentative steps in the Affordable Care Act in things such as accountable care organizations, the Independent Payment Advisory Board, and various grants for pilot programs and information systems. These will all seek to, in Washington speak, "bend the cost curve." But when you're in a boat that is taking on water fast and may sink, you don't try to "bend the curve" of how much water is coming in; you try to plug the hole and start bailing. The cost control provisions of the Affordable Care Act don't plug the hole we already have, punch a few new ones for good measure, and bail with a paper cup.

Growing bureaucracy and control

Government loves complexity, rules, and red tape, but we may have outdone ourselves this time. Reform offered a chance to clean up the baroque system we have created over the years, reduce bureaucracy, lower administrative cost, and give clarity and focus to a major part of where we spend our taxpayer's money. Instead, we created yet more complexity, more regulations, and the need for more bureaucracy.

Let's do a thought experiment: imagine that our current Congress is transported back in time to the mid-1930s. We're in the midst of the Depression and there's a movement to ensure that the elderly have basic financial security. FDR calls on our time-transported 111th Congress to solve this problem; he asks them for an Elderly Protection and Affordable Living Act that he can sign. They've just finished their 418,000–word health reform effort and are ready to go to work.

Here's how our Congress from the year 2010 would approach it. The first order of business would be to mandate that every American be required to have a pension plan; if you don't, you'll pay a fine. The federal government will decide how extensive your pension plan needs to be: they'll decide what's appropriate for you. Next, this time-traveling Congress will place on your employer the obligation to offer you such a pension plan or pay fines. There are lots of exemptions for hundreds of thousands of smaller businesses; there are subsidies for others. Since many Americans won't be able to afford their now legally required pension plan, the Congress will set up a complicated set of subsidies that depend on income and family circumstances. They'll set up a large bureaucracy to administer those subsidies. The subsidy will vary from year to year as each person's income and situation changes. Then they'll set up an Exchange to link up these subsidized citizens with an approved list of pension plans. If you've had to accept the government's subsidy to meet your mandate requirement, you'll be subject to rules on some things you *have* to spend your retirement money on, and some things you *can't*.

Fortunately, the 74th Congress chose a less rococo approach. They passed a simple payroll tax, equally shared by employer and employee. The revenues from this tax were routed through a trust fund, which then issued monthly checks to the elderly to use as they saw fit. It took them 15,600 words. We call it Social Security.

Finances that are too clever

In the conduct of America's affairs, elected officials embrace many different values and approach problems from different ideological points of view. For our government to work, however, these debates should be conducted against the background of an honest and conservative evaluation of their financial effects. This is true whether the subject is Republicans proposing tax cuts or Democrats talking about the expansion of social programs. The Affordable Care Act doesn't measure up to that standard.

The CBO is an independent arm of Congress with very capable people and a long tradition of objective analysis. But they work within the framework of a set of rules that sometimes conceal the underlying realities. In their "scoring" of the Affordable Care Act, for example, one of the significant ways of paying for expanding health insurance coverage was the use of premiums from the new CLASS Act entitlement that was established. The legislation begins collecting premiums for this insurance in 2015, but doesn't begin paying out benefits until 2020 (conveniently, here in 2010, just outside of the CBO ten-year time horizon). The CBO "scoring" of the legislation takes those first five years of premiums and diverts them to paying for its expansion of coverage. This diversion represents $70 billion of the offsets to the costs of the legislation. It assumes that when it becomes necessary to begin paying benefits in 2020, there will be other premiums from other Americans to cover the cost. When an insurance company in Tennessee (and I presume the other forty-nine states as well) occasionally does this—collects insurance premiums and diverts them elsewhere, planning to pay claims later with other premiums—we shut them down.

In addition, during the debate on the Affordable Care Act, a great many people observed that some of the savings being claimed were very questionable. In particular, the CBO analysis took credit for $198 billion of savings from reducing Medicare provider rates in future years. Since Congress has been unable since 2002 to allow a previous rate reduction to occur, some skepticism is in order.

Every business executive knows that in an analysis like this, the costs are certain and they start on Monday morning without fail. The revenues and savings that are designed to pay those costs always balance nicely in the spreadsheets, but are far less certain in the world. Tennessee got in deep trouble with its Medicaid expansion in the early 1990s for precisely that reason; we proved to ourselves it would work on paper, but when we added lots of real people, the costs came in on schedule, and the savings didn't. The Affordable Care Act has this exact vulnerability.

The passage of the Affordable Care Act was made politically acceptable by setting up a straw man: would it reduce the deficit or not? When the CBO announced that the legislation would indeed reduce it, the political path to passage was cleared. But if we make even the most obvious and sensible real-world adjustments to their analysis, the answer is different. Take out the CLASS Act funds—no insurance company in America would be allowed to do what the CBO rules permitted. Add an estimate of the real cost of appropriations that were made for one year but clearly intended to be continued, and include an estimate of the new administrative costs in HHS and the IRS. In May, well after the Affordable Care Acts's passage, the CBO added an additional $115 billion to the cost of the legislation to reflect these. Add an estimate for the appropriations for which there were no numbers, only "sum sufficient" language. These are not esoteric adjustments, just commonsense ones. But when they're made, the legislation no longer "reduces the deficit," it adds to it. If you don't believe the Medicare rate reductions will actually happen, it adds even more.

Knocking over a straw man with CBO rules was good politics and similar bits of theater have been used often by Republicans as well. But I expected more of my party. Congress and the president made much of requiring "transparency" in all things health care;

some of that same transparency in the ways we're paying for this legislation would have been appropriate.

The retreat from post-partisanship

There's an old saying that if the only tool you have is a hammer, you make every problem into a nail. In our political process, if the only tool we have—or choose to use—is the game of partisan competition, then we force every problem in our society to be played out on a Republican–Democrat axis and solved in those terms. America has always had ideological differences, but problems like those surrounding our health care system are complex and multidimensional. The dynamics of partisan politics in Washington collapses these issues into a single dimension, but out here in the rest of the country, the world feels richer and more multidimensional than that.

At the beginning of 2009, there were a lot of Americans from many political camps who believed that Barack Obama was the man to start breaking down this dysfunctional partisanship. I was one of them, and was optimistic that he'd work to return us to a style of governance that remained competitive but was far more collegial and focused on results. That was one of his promises and health reform had great possibility as a vehicle for this. The desire to reduce the ranks of the uninsured is genuinely bipartisan. Some of the boldest plans for doing so have come from Republican governors in places like Massachusetts and California. The largest expansion of any social program in decades—the Medicare Part D Program, which subsidized the cost of prescription drugs for Medicare beneficiaries—was the work of a Republican Congress in 2003. Here, with a new president who promised a post-partisan era, was the chance to start.

Instead, the president left the design of his reform to the most partisan body in America. Democrats were firmly in the majority and wrote the legislation, and the dream of beginning a new post-partisan era came down to the chairman of the Senate Finance

Committee trying to find a few tweaks that might dress up the final vote with a Republican senator or two. Once that was over, bipartisanship was pronounced dead and Congress and the president returned without further ado to business as usual. It was as if a band of pioneers had set out in their covered wagons for Oregon, found a modest hill they'd have to surmount in Missouri, thrown up their hands, turned around, and gone back home.

We have health care reform legislation now, but we didn't use the opportunity it presented as a way to begin fixing our political process. Instead, if anything, we opened the wounds wider. It's possible to accumulate power by dividing people, by driving wedges, and exaggerating differences. But leadership is about finding common ground and moving forward. We've usually managed to do that in our country when the issues were large. We don't go to war on tight, party-line votes. Dan Balz of the *Washington Post* has pointed out that other major social legislation, while contentious, ultimately passed with strong bipartisan majorities. Social Security passed the House in 1935 with a vote of 372–77; it passed the Senate 77–6. In both cases, a majority of the Republicans voted for the measure. Medicare was approved in 1965 by the House on a 313–115 vote and the Senate on a 68–21 vote; in each body, about half of the Republicans voted for the measure.

Perhaps I'm mistaken and perhaps our president was right when he called the vote on health reform answering "the call of history." I believe something different though: that if we listen carefully to the call of history, it asks us to do the big things together. It's an odd place for this president to be. I'd expect a man with roots in "community organizing" to harbor a deep trust for the values and sensibility of ordinary Americans and a distrust of the powerful institutions of our society. But health reform has been just the opposite: an insider's game in Washington, influenced by powerful institutions, and pushed through with some very hard-nosed politics over what appears to be widespread and deep concern among those ordinary Americans. It's always dangerous to believe that you know best what's really good for someone else, even if they don't agree. I predict that we're a long way from counting all the costs of a 219–212 House vote—with no Republicans—on health reform.

The mandate and the Constitution

My final reservation is not strictly about health care, and it's more a reservation I want to express than an outright criticism. The federal mandate that requires the purchase of health insurance is a new feature on the American landscape and those who express concern about it as an unjustified extension of federal power deserve a careful hearing. Tennessee didn't join the states filing lawsuits over the constitutionality of this aspect of the Affordable Care Act. I consulted with a number of people who know something about constitutional law and didn't have an ideological view of the Affordable Care Act. On the whole, their advice was that they believed the mandate, and the tax assessment for those who fail to comply with it, fit within the scope of federal authority as it's been worked out in the Supreme Court over the years. Furthermore, the lawsuits had a highly partisan feel about them; perhaps the Republican legislators showing the most outrage on this particular occasion had forgotten that their colleagues had proposed exactly the same thing back in 1993 as an alternative to the Clinton reforms.

The mandate may well prove to be constitutional, but it does give a lot of reasonable people indigestion. During my lifetime, the issues relating to the extent of constitutional federal authority have been expressed in unfortunate contexts. For most of the past half century, "states' rights" has been a synonym for segregation. As I write this, the issues are being raised most vocally by so-called "tea-party" members, whose rhetoric couples this legitimate issue with too many distinctly over-the-top ones.

It's unfortunate this has happened. Our nation benefits from the energy of distinct state and federal powers in the same way that it benefits from the separation of powers among the three branches of our national government. As a governor, I believe that the states have a separate and important role to play in the conduct of our nation's affairs. They are surely more than a subordinate administrative arm of the federal government. But if this is the case, it implies that there are limitations to the domain of the federal government.

The federal government clearly has the power to levy taxes. I have no objection to Social Security in this regard, nor, as you'll see later, any objection to doing the same for health care. But the mandate's negative space approach—compelling an individual to do something by taxing the absence of it—represents a new dimension. If the mandate can be justified constitutionally because it has a relationship to economic activity (what doesn't) and therefore falls under the Commerce Clause, or even more fundamentally, simply as the power to tax, it's hard to see that there remain any real constitutional limitations to federal power.

In his speech to Congress in September 2009, President Obama declared, "I am not the first president to take up this cause, but I am determined to be the last." I listened to that speech and I believe he was completely sincere. But he *won't* be the last, because so many underlying problems of financial sustainability were not only ignored but, if anything, made worse. Making it possible for tens of millions of people to have health insurance who are without it today is a very good thing, but doing it by adding them to an already unsustainable system just kicks the can down the road a bit farther. There's a very difficult problem awaiting some future president.

When we step back and look at the Affordable Care Act in the largest terms, at its core it's a victory for the economic interests of those who supply health care. It expanded coverage, producing more revenues. The industry in the best position to bargain—the health insurance industry—was made the enemy and weakened.

In the 2010 Fortune 500 listings, all eleven of the health insurance and managed care companies taken together had less profit than a single pharmaceutical company: Merck (profits of $12.9 billion, a 47% after-tax margin on their revenues). With the Affordable Care Act, we've pushed the insurance industry to become more like a simple utility, designed to quietly and efficiently pass money, without asking too many questions, from taxpayers and businesses to the health care industry.

We've been in places like this before. In the final decades of the nineteenth century, the industrial revolution drove tremendous growth in the American economy—this was the age of steel mills and railroads. The corporate wealth it produced was visible and powerful, but a long list of problems was developing in the shadows. That image of a golden veneer of wealth obscuring a base metal of growing problems is what gave the time its label: the Gilded Age. It was followed by the Progressive Era, when the excesses of those decades were curtailed and broader public interests addressed.

Just as the industrial revolution drove our economy then, the scientific revolution has driven it in the final decades of the twentieth century. In few places is that more evident than health care; in 1960 per capita health care expenditures were $1,100 (in 2010 dollars), today they're over $8,000 and rising rapidly. The railroad and steel companies of the Gilded Age have been replaced by ones that make pharmaceuticals and medical devices. But the pattern is familiar.

Once again we need real reform, but I would respectfully suggest that the game we've just played is as old as politics itself. Even when the demand for change gets loud, political figures have known for a long time that its possible to still protect the status quo and keep your friends. You just spruce it up with some new clothes and a little lipstick and *call* it reformed. When we begin our reform with a backroom deal promising the pharmaceutical industry that we'll leave them alone for years to come, it would be wise to wipe off the lipstick and take a careful look.

3

The Roots of America's Health Care System

... in which we consider how medical care has evolved over the years and how its history has shaped the structure of today's American health care system.

Throughout human history, we've placed a very high value on the health of our bodies. It's a primal urge—evolution has wired a drive for self-preservation and well-being into our brains. We want to live long lives, we want to enjoy capable bodies, and we want to avoid pain and suffering. When we're injured, we want to be healed. When we contract disease, we want to be cured. If we can't be cured, we want our suffering reduced. We want delay and then succor for the inevitable pains of aging and death. We want these things for ourselves and for our friends and loved ones as well.

As a result, throughout human history, healing has been a priority of human societies and healers have enjoyed a privileged place in them. Ancient Egypt had an extensive system of physicians (including specialists such as ophthalmologists and dentists) and the best of them were highly valued. Ancient Greece is partially remembered by the work of Hippocrates to codify and extend medical knowledge; physicians marched with armies in ancient Rome and developed battle-tested remedies that remain appropriate even today. The best evidence of the high value societies have placed on healing comes from its central place in many religious practices. Primitive societies often assigned a religious or spiritual function to those whom they believed could heal injuries or cure disease. When Christ set out to prove his divinity, he frequently did so by healing the afflicted—a leper, a centurion's servant afflicted by palsy, a man with a shriveled hand, an invalid who could not walk, a man born blind. The importance of healing and healers is a thread that has run through human societies throughout our history. I imagine that if I could visit an ancient village of Neanderthals, a man or woman who was believed to have the power to heal would be an important figure. In America right now, being able to say that you're a doctor confers immediate respect and deference.

The pace of change

While the importance of medicine has been a thread that runs throughout our history, it's taken on a different level of importance in our modern world. The explosion of scientific knowledge that has dominated human history in the twentieth century has had a profound impact on the practice of medicine. For example, societies going back at least five millennia have had herbal formularies, but with the scientific revolution came the isolation and understanding of the chemicals in those herbs that produced their effects. That allowed us to isolate and purify them and to experiment with variations. Other scientific advances helped us understand the biochemical mechanisms underlying their actions and, with that knowledge, to invent new ways of accomplishing the same thing. Many of the drugs in a modern pharmacy trace their roots to the lore of ancient herbalists, but their modern incarnations are far safer and more potent.

At the beginning of the twentieth century, the medical revolution was just getting underway. Louis Pasteur and Joseph Lister had helped us understand where disease came from, and many of the infectious agents that had plagued mankind were now being identified. X-rays had just been discovered and instruments that would serve medicine—to measure blood pressure, for example— were being invented. Surgery was becoming much safer with the employment of anesthetics and knowledge about how to prevent infection. Yet a great many infectious diseases were still dangerous, and medical events that would be trivial in the decades ahead still claimed lives. Diagnosed and treated in time, appendicitis is cured with a modest and safe operation today. Not much more than a century ago it was a life-threatening event.

These changes have taken place quickly, very much within the memory of living people. I grew up with my grandmother, who was born in the last decade of the nineteenth century. I remember a conversation with her one day about medicine. It was on her mind as she was getting older and she wanted me to understand how different it had been in her youth. I sat in our living room—it was the late 1960s—and tried to imagine as she talked about a very different world, alien to me but still very familiar to her. It was a world with few medical X-rays and no antibiotics; one in which infectious diseases were still a common scourge. She told me about the very real fear every parent had of losing a child to disease. In the 1930s, it happened to her, and she lost a beautiful sixteen-year-old daughter to an illness that would be treated today with an inexpensive antibiotic. All the years I lived with her, she didn't permit the word "polio" to be spoken in our house because it still had fearsome connotations. It was in the same forbidden category as playing "Taps" on my school band trumpet. Perhaps one of my descendants will someday tell their own grandchildren of a time when the word "cancer" conjured up those same fears. The young twenty-second century listeners will struggle just a little to envision that world, such is the pace of progress in the science of medicine.

The power of medicine has grown exponentially in the past century, from the world of my grandmother's youth without X-rays to one today with MRI scans, organ transplants, and genetic screening. Along with scientific advances, there have been other changes. One very visible one is that medical care costs more, a lot more. Before we immerse ourselves in statistics of percentages of GDP devoted to health care, consider a simple real-world example. In 1900, an early form of health insurance was provided by a large array of fraternal societies. Among the services they might offer their members was a primitive form of health insurance called "lodge practice." The cost of an annual contract for this early form of health insurance was about a day's wage for a typical laborer. Today, that same typical laborer would pay about two month's wages for a typical health insurance plan for just himself. To be fair, a modern worker's plan covers many more things, but that's a part of the story as well.

A less obvious change, but just as far-reaching, is how much the complexity of actually delivering medical care has grown. Medicine is no longer just a doctor and a patient. There have long been specialists for certain kinds of illnesses, but even a century ago much of medical care was still a one-on-one relationship between a patient and a physician. Today, even common illnesses often involve multiple physicians and bringing to bear a wide variety of other medical services. One factor causing this new complexity is increasing specialization and subspecialization among physicians. Some of this is a natural result of the growth in knowledge about treating disease and some is the equally natural result of the value our society places on this specialization. We demonstrate that value by our willingness to compensate those with this specialized knowledge very well.

But much of this new complexity is just the result of the array of technological resources that are brought to bear on even simple illnesses: highly technical laboratory work, for example, and complex imaging services that range from modern versions of venerable X-rays to CT scanners and MRI devices. This growth in complexity has been going on for a long time and is an important feature of health care in America today. One indication is the high priority we've placed on health information systems and electronic health records. These are a staple of "good government" in health care and have been mandated and funded extensively by the Obama administration. These information systems are largely just a way to try to deal with this growing complexity. It's common for even quite healthy individuals to interact with the health care system in many separate ways over the course of a year—emergency rooms, primary care doctors, specialists, outpatient services, perhaps even a hospital stay. With this complexity, there's an obvious need to consolidate the resulting information in one place so that a patient can receive care that's as coordinated as possible. Good information systems are the foundation for accomplishing this. We'll discuss later how we might stimulate demand from providers for these, rather than pushing these systems on them with incentives and penalties. However it's accomplished, much better use of information systems is a vital part of the response to the growing complexity of medical care.

The early history of reform

Over the past century, as the costs and complexity of health care have grown, there have been several efforts in the public sector to expand its reach and alter the payment arrangements—efforts at "reform." To be fair, while I've been critical of the Affordable Care Act for being concerned primarily with expanding access, that approach is consistent with what "reform" has been about in the past. That history doesn't excuse the serious failure of the Affordable Care Act to address major issues confronting us (such as cost and sustainability), but perhaps makes it more understandable.

Something resembling what we consider health insurance came into being at the very end of the nineteenth century. In an era where industrial work was often dangerous, insurance companies offered policies to protect against accidental injury or death. It was a natural extension to broaden these policies to cover specific diseases, and then to broaden them further to cover disabilities that resulted from either disease or accident. These policies provided a way to pay for the medical costs of an illness, but were even more a form of income security. The interest in government-provided social insurance was far less in America than in Europe, possibly reflecting both the decentralized nature of American government and its political stability—there was less of a political imperative to satisfy workers here.

The first big push for government involvement in the financing of health insurance came during World War I, when the American Association for Labor Legislation (AALL) proposed and worked for health insurance for working-class Americans. They ran into several roadblocks. President Woodrow Wilson didn't engage, and so this attempt didn't have a driving force at high levels of government. Many in the labor movement didn't support it, most particularly Samuel Gompers of the American Federation of Labor. In his view, extracting this benefit on behalf of labor was the role of unions and when done by government was paternalistic and ultimately demeaning to workers. He opposed government action to set a minimum wage and establish an eight-hour work day on similar grounds. Combined with this labor opposition, physicians were loath to support any effort that would place any party in a position from which they could negotiate fees or any other conditions of their practice. While presidents came and went, and most of labor altered its view, physicians drew a line in the sand that remained a barrier for decades. (Interestingly, one of the arguments made by reformers was that broad and secure health insurance would encourage preventive care. Another was that broad and compulsory insurance would eliminate the overhead and profits of the insurance industry, and that the cost of the expansion could be substantially financed in this way. The more things change . . .)

Two decades later, during the Great Depression, economic conditions and the advent of the New Deal renewed interest in social insurance. Physicians by this time were clear and united in a protectionist view of their profession and the American Medical Association was strong and well-organized. FDR, however, was lukewarm in his support—he was reluctant to take on organized medicine— and ultimately instead placed his political chips on the square of old-age economic security—Social Security—rather than health reform.

While the federal government again declined to play a comprehensive role, the 1930s did see the creation of what we think of today as health insurance. Medical care was steadily becoming more expensive and the economic concern of Americans was shifting away from the need for income security during an illness to the need for a way to pay for the costs of the illness itself. The progenitor of what we now call Blue Cross was an insurance policy developed by Justin Ford Kimball and offered by Baylor University Hospital in 1929. The hospital offered teachers up to twenty-one days of hospital care in their hospital for an annual fee of $6. Other individual hospitals followed suit. About three years later, the concept was extended to include all of a community's hospitals and not just a single one.

The intimate connection of this new form of insurance with the hospitals themselves led to a feature that helped the insurance to grow rapidly. Because the insurance risk could be passed on to the hospital—they would agree to provide the service regardless of their compensation—it took very little capital to start one of these plans. The hospitals' guarantees served as the capital of the insurance firms (very much like what would happen a half century later with the expansion of the HMO industry). In many cases, these insurance plans were started with a few thousand dollars in capital. These "Blue Cross" plans that offered services at all the hospitals within a community were more attractive to the public than the single-hospital plans, and throughout the 1930s continued to grow. As nonprofits, and because of their intimate links with hospitals, they had a financial advantage over commercial insurance and dominated the new health industry increasingly as time went on. Physicians permitted these arrangements as long as there was no attempt to include any physician payments in the system.

At the same time, the National Labor Relations Act in 1935 required management to bargain with labor over the terms and conditions of employment. Many unions had been reluctant to offer health benefits to their members, feeling that the increases in dues that would be required would interfere with the growth of union membership. But now health benefits were a legitimate target of negotiation and the era of employer-provided health insurance, still with us, was born. The number of Americans who had health insurance exploded in the years ahead, from less than 10% of the population in 1940 to nearly 70% fifteen years later.

Many of the important features of our health insurance system today trace their lineage to the events of a relatively short span of time during the 1930s. Today's structure of medical payments as "insurance" grows out of the fact that that's how the first really successful payment system began—as insurance against an unexpected hospitalization. The separation of payments for physician services from other parts of health care traces its roots back to the political arrangement that permitted the Blue Cross insurance plans to conduct their business. The dominance of employer-based insurance today is a consequence of both FDR's backing away from a government role and the passage of the National Labor Relations Act, making health insurance coverage an achievable goal for unions. In the 1930s, the provision of this particular form of social insurance—health insurance—became firmly privatized, where it substantially remains today.

After World War II

Almost immediately after the end of the Second World War, President Truman took up the cause once again of a national health insurance system. The Truman plan was the first to propose a single health insurance system for everyone, rather than a separate system for the needy. It was vehemently opposed by the American Medical Association (AMA) and at the beginning of the Cold War era it was easy to label such a plan a socialist plot and turn opinion against it. When Republicans won control of Congress in 1946, it was effectively dead. Truman ran for reelection promising national health insurance, but the time had passed, public sentiment had turned against it, and other issues such as the Korean War took center stage.

While President Truman's concept of universal coverage was dead, administrators in the Social Security program and elsewhere continued work on the idea of health insurance specifically for beneficiaries of the Social Security system. This ultimately resulted in the Social Security Act of 1965, which established Medicare. President Johnson signed it into law on July 30, 1965, and Harry S. Truman was enrolled and presented with the first Medicare card. This began the modern era of government support of health insurance for broad populations.

As a brief review: Medicare is health insurance that is universal to everyone over the age of sixty-five. It began with two components. The first, Medicare Part A, is hospital insurance and is paid for by a payroll tax. This Medicare Part A tax essentially adds an additional 2.9% to the Social Security tax: 1.45% from the employee and another 1.45% from the employer. These taxes are paid into a trust fund and Medicare Part A is self-financing: the payroll taxes pay for the benefits received. (The Affordable Care Act extends the payroll tax to higher incomes and adds an additional tax on investment income as well.) Medicare Part B is medical insurance, as opposed to hospital insurance, and pays for physician services, laboratory tests, hospital outpatient procedures, and medical equipment such as wheelchairs and prosthetic devices, and a variety of similar items. It's partially funded by a Part B monthly premium paid by those who belong to the Medicare system, and partially by general government revenues.

Much later, in 2003, Medicare Part D to pay for prescription drugs was added; it's partially funded by a premium paid by the Medicare beneficiary and partially by general tax revenues. In 2010, Medicare Part D was expanded further in the Affordable Care Act; this was the so-called "closing the donut hole."

The Social Security Act of 1965 also created the Medicaid program. This was originally designed to be health insurance for poor women, their children, and the disabled, although it has been extended far beyond that original group over the years. Today, fifty-eight million Americans (19% of the population) receive their health care through Medicaid. In my state of Tennessee, Medicaid covers more than 1.4 million people (23% of the population) and pays over $7 billion for health care annually. Under the Affordable Care Act, Medicaid will expand by another eighteen million people. Medicaid is a joint responsibility of the federal government and the states, with the federal government paying on average about 57% of its costs and the states 43%; states provide the administration of the program. The actual split in financial responsibility varies from state to state based on a state's level of personal income. The wealthiest states, such as California, Minnesota, or New Hampshire pay the legal state maximum share of 50%. The poorest state, Mississippi, pays about 24% of its Medicaid costs. This ratio of federal to state participation in paying for the program is known by the acronym FMAP (Federal Medical Assistance Percentages) and has been widely discussed in the context of the stimulus plan as a vehicle for the federal government to deliver financial assistance to the states during the current recession.

I obviously have no personal memory of the earlier attempts at what we now term health care reform—I've only read about them—but I do remember very well the passage of the Medicare and Medicaid legislation in 1965. I was a college student at the time, thought it was all wonderful, and was absolutely convinced that universal health care was now just around the corner, a matter of a few years at most. I also remember vividly how much many of the health professionals hated it, especially Medicare. I had worked in our local small-town drug store when I was in high school, and still visited my old boss when I came home during college breaks. He was convinced that Medicare proved that the Communists had finally won. Our differing views actually became a real barrier between two people who liked each other and had spent a lot of evenings in the drug store together. I didn't know the general practitioner in our town very well, but the reaction of my pharmacist boss's was mild in comparison to his.

And yet, although there was certainly strong opposition to the Medicare Act from some parts of the medical community, the expansions of government involvement in access to care, in the end, were accepted more easily this time. The long-standing hostility of the medical profession to any party they thought would have the power to negotiate terms with them was a moot point by then. They were defending a position that had already been lost—many of their patients now had health insurance written by companies doing just that. While Medicare offended a long-held view of what a physician's economic relationship with his patients should be, it also offered the promise of a comfortable income.

The "silver bullet" view of medicine

As I've already noted, for a long time now the public discussion of health care has revolved around expanding access to it. But, more quietly, other changes have been taking place that have had a profound effect on the structure of health care today. One of them has been our increasing fascination with sophisticated technology as the fundamental building block of medicine.

After the end of the Second World War, this view came naturally. Science had won the war and ushered in the atomic age. America was a land of televisions, jet airplanes, and room-filling computers churning out answers. Could an idealized world of airplane cars and automatic kitchens be far behind? I remember the decade of the fifties well; I graduated from high school as it concluded. The ethos was clear: we were to apply scientific principles to problems in every sphere and the solutions were there waiting for our discovery. It's natural that this ethic would be applied to medicine as well.

There's a great deal of truth in that view, and scientific advances have improved the effectiveness of medicine and will continue to do so indefinitely. But in most areas of life we have a more nuanced view today—we've outgrown the infatuation of the fifties and sixties in which science and technology held all the answers. Our view of medical care, however, is still a throwback to that era. We still embrace a "silver bullet" view of medicine—that for every problem, there's a wonder drug or a new treatment that's either in our arsenal or just waiting to be discovered. We're fascinated by and place too much reliance on technology. I remember going to a doctor (not my current one) for a physical many years ago. I was approaching middle age and my cholesterol was starting to creep up. He wanted me to start taking one of the cholesterol-lowering drugs: Lipitor. His argument was this: relax, there's no reason why you shouldn't eat cheeseburgers if you want, now there's a pill that will fix the cholesterol problem. He didn't say so, but I assume he also had in mind that even if I did clog up my arteries, there were always more drugs and plenty of surgeons ready to do a coronary bypass. (Fortunately, I listened to my wife instead and lightened up on the french fries.)

Even at the end of life, when the most natural of processes is underway, we often continue to cling to a belief in those silver bullets in the hope that science and technology can in some way hold back death. Long life is a highly desirable and valued product of medical care. But placing too much emphasis on it, as any medical practitioner can tell you often happens, becomes bizarre and robs death of the dignity that has been valued throughout human history.

This fascination with complex technological solutions distorts where we place our trust and resources in medicine. The use of technology by its very nature tends to happen well along in the progression of a disease, and it often takes place in a complex setting such as a hospital or a specialist's office. A lot of resources are consumed there and the technology used is expensive. What's shortchanged by this emphasis is investment in the earlier and lower-tech parts of medicine: investments that are not so spectacular but more productive.

If someone is unfortunate enough to be diagnosed with colorectal cancer, there's a vast array of technology available to try to save them. But what really determines their chances is how far the disease has progressed before its discovery. That person might well have been better served if our health care system put more of its resources into this early detection rather than trying to fix things later.

A part of our cost problem in health care is the uncritical view we take of all this new technology. We take it as an article of faith that we should, as a matter of moral obligation, find a way to pay for every new drug, every new surgery, every new technology, every "breakthrough." Real scientific advances in medicine need to be quickly disseminated and used, but we have to begin with being selective and critical in our evaluation and rejecting the notion that every new thing in medicine that can claim science in its parentage is instantly embraced.

Medicine has always been part magic. It deals with life and death. It's power flows from a vast body of arcane knowledge. Science and technology have become the new magic, with powers both real and imagined. There are a lot of people today who make a fine living out of that magic and are unlikely to be critical. A part of our job with health care today is to find ways to look under the surface. We need to embrace the real magic—and there's plenty of it—but be selective and not put our faith and resources where they don't belong. Doing a thorough checkup or helping someone with their obesity may be less magical than doing an MRI or bypass surgery, but in the end, much more important.

What we mean by "health care"

Another quiet but profound change in health care has been the steady expansion of what we consider its role to be. Some of that expansion is natural and reflects our increased prosperity; medical conditions representing the commonplace illnesses of life and that once passed unremarked are now treated by professionals. Childhood infectious diseases, colds, sore throats, the flu, the aches and pains and stresses of just being alive are all well-represented in emergency rooms and doctor's offices, right along with broken bones and heart attacks.

In the 1950s and '60s, social reformers saw medicine as the scientific approach to a host of societal problems that had formerly been dealt with in other ways. We've had substance abusers and deviant behavior for a long time. For most of that time those conditions have been treated as moral failings and punitive measures were considered the proper response. But with the faith that science could provide solutions here as well, a range of behavioral issues moved from being considered a part of the fabric of society firmly into the domain of medicine, where they reside today. Although the science is much softer in these areas—diagnosis is inconsistent and there are fewer rigorous standards for treatment—mental health is achieving parity with the rest of medicine and represents a real extension of its domain. Let me be clear that I don't object to that— these conditions are real and deeply impact the lives of people who are afflicted with them. If medicine and science can offer solutions, humanity benefits. But it opens an entirely new landscape in medical care and expands its responsibilities a great deal.

In a similar fashion, there are many conditions that are likely encompassed comfortably in the normal range of human variation that we now consider something to be treated medically. We've assumed a narrow definition of what's "normal." This is evident, for example, in the rapidly growing diagnosis and treatment of various behaviors in children. ADHD (Attention-Deficit Hyperactivity Disorder) is now widely diagnosed and treated. I don't doubt that there are genuine behaviors being observed, but the indications for diagnosing ADHD (not paying attention to details, making careless mistakes in homework, failing to finish schoolwork and chores, not wanting to do things that take a lot of mental effort for a long period of time, and so on) are commonplace and in many cases may fall well within the range of how ordinary human children act.

As our population ages, the medical issues that come with age become more and more prevalent. These were seen not too long ago as natural—a part of the aging process. Today, the ethic is different: much of this is clearly defined as a disease that commands aggressive treatment. There's nothing inherently wrong with this; medicine has been looked to for a long time to ameliorate the pains and disease of old age. But in its extent, it is once again an expansion of the domain of health care.

Finally, in our affluent society, we increasingly demand access to medical care that is essentially reassuring in nature. Checkups and prevention have assumed a much more central role in our medical system and are strongly encouraged—mandated, in fact—in the Affordable Care Act. Some of this is well-justified on medical grounds, but less than you might think. Much of it is simply about assuring the healthy that they're okay.

This expansion of the domain of what's considered health care isn't inherently bad, but we have to be careful about the meanings of words here. We're naming a large, growing, and casually selected collection of services "health care." When we then use that same term to describe those things to which we seek to guarantee access as a moral right of citizens, we go astray. We're being sloppy and inconsistent in our definition of "health care"—not everything grouped under that term carries the same moral weight. If someone has appendicitis, of course they're entitled to treatment. We're going to take care of pregnant women and ensure healthy babies as a moral obligation. But anytime I turn on the television in the evening, I can see ads for prescription pharmaceuticals—expensive ones—whose purpose is to help the attractive woman in the commercial get a good night's sleep. That woman should be allowed to buy that medication if that's how she wants to conduct her life. But I don't feel any moral obligation to take money from someone else through taxes to pay for it for her.

Looking ahead for a moment, one of the difficult jobs realistically awaiting us as a nation will be to separate all those things that have come to be lumped together as health care into two categories. One will be the core services that are truly important to health and well-being and should be guaranteed as a right to all. The other will be a large and growing halo of other kinds of health care that may well be useful and desirable, but don't rise to the level of a moral obligation. Removing an infected appendix and providing excellent prenatal care for a pregnant woman are in the first category; expensive sleeping pills are in the second.

4

Health "Insurance"

. . . in which we look more closely at one of our health care system's relics from an earlier time—the reliance on an insurance paradigm as the way to pay for medical care. We see that it's inefficient, rewards the wrong behavior, and that abandoning it will be essential for real reform.

There are many features of today's health care system that have their roots in its history. There's one, however, that stands out from all others as a fundamental source of many of its problems—the continued reliance on an insurance model for paying for health care. We're on the wrong road; somewhere along the way we missed the turnoff.

We call it "health insurance," but it isn't. Insurance is an old and well-established concept. It's characterized by protecting the insured against unusual and well-defined events. In concept, it works like this: imagine a town with a thousand houses, and in any year the chances are that one of them might burn down. An insurance company collects a premium of one one-thousandth of the value of a house from everyone. If it's your house that burns down, you collect the money to rebuild it. If it's not your house, you consider yourself lucky and the benefit you get from paying the insurance premium is the security and peace of mind that results. The house fire is a rare event, it takes place at a specific point in time, the payment the homeowner who bought the insurance receives is well-defined—it's either an agreed-upon cost to repair the damage or the value of the home.

As we've just discussed in the previous chapter, decades ago health insurance was real insurance. It was narrowly designed to protect against the unforeseen costs of an unexpected illness or injury. Remember the early origins of the modern Blue Cross system in that Texas hospital that sold a very precise insurance policy: if you unexpectedly needed hospital care, it paid for twenty-one days in that specific hospital. Period. For a long time, health insurance was focused primarily on paying the costs of an unexpected hospital stay. Even today, "hospitalization" remains a synonym for "health insurance" with many older Americans.

That's not how it works any more. There are still genuine insurance aspects to a policy—you might have an accident or contract an unexpected disease. But vast amounts of the money that flows through our health system looks nothing like an insurance transaction. Rather than the unexpected, a great deal of what is paid for is completely expected. We use our health insurance for preventive care and checkups, for common illnesses like the flu, for prescriptions that we may take for years for our high blood pressure or high cholesterol. Chronic illnesses such as diabetes and heart disease are characterized by open-ended expenses that may occur every month over a period of years or even decades. The expenses that many of us will incur in the later years of life are significant and may occur over a relatively short period of time, but are hardly unexpected. These are completely appropriate expenditures, and there's a need to budget them properly so that we can pay for medical care when it's needed, but it no longer looks anything like real insurance. Yet we continue to think of it in terms of an insurance model: we call it "insurance," we pay "premiums," and our doctor submits a "claim" for her services.

Let's do a thought experiment. Imagine for a moment that our home owner's insurance had evolved to work like health insurance does today. Perhaps Blue Cross had decided back in the 1930s to get into the field of insuring people's homes against damage as well as insuring their health. There would today be a nationwide Blue Hammer organization that provides homeowner insurance for millions of Americans. If there were a big unexpected event—let's say a fire—Blue Hammer would pay to have your house repaired. But instead of settling your claim with you, instead it would directly pay a myriad of individual claims from many different contractors who didn't necessarily coordinate with one another on the repairs. It would pay for whatever those contractors deemed in their judgment was needed, with no overall management of the total cost or quality of the repairs. Furthermore, Blue Hammer insurance would also cover many of the things we'd consider normal maintenance: if the house needed painting, or the steps repaired, or you wanted the floors refinished, that would be covered by your insurance as well. The contractors you would deal with would recommend things they believed should be done to your home (and which were incidentally also quite profitable to them). If you agreed, the work would be done, the bill would go to Blue Hammer, and you likely wouldn't even know the cost.

Anyone can see intuitively that this would be very expensive and inefficient insurance indeed. There are few people who'd wish to pay for this version of home owner's insurance out of their own pocket. If it were the responsibility of their employer or the government, that might be a different matter.

Our continued attempt to dress the way we pay for health care in the garments of the insurance industry clouds our thinking about it and is at the root of much that we know needs changing. There are few things that people criticize more frequently when it comes to waste in health spending than the amount of administrative overhead involved. There's indeed far too much overhead, but the enemy isn't insurance companies, it's insurance itself.

In our medical care system, this continued reliance on paying for individual medical services as separate insurance claims produces an astonishing amount of paperwork and overhead. Even when I visit my doctor for the simplest and least-expensive of reasons—an annual physical, for example—the behind-the-scenes mechanics for my doctor to get paid are astonishing. On the day of my visit, he'll fill out an encounter form, which details a number of individual services that will constitute my physical. For this routine visit, these might include his own consultation with me, some lab tests, a chest X-ray, and an electrocardiogram. After he's has done this, a coding specialist will likely check it and then the codes describing each of these separate services are entered individually into a computer by a data entry person in the physician's office. A bill is then prepared detailing all this and forwarded to an outside company which in turn submits it electronically to my own insurance company. My insurance company will be one of perhaps a hundred that a large practice deals with.

When it arrives at the insurance company, that bill for my annual physical is audited in a variety of ways. Most insurance companies have a number of so-called "black box" audits of the charges that are submitted. They might check, for example, whether the complexity of the visit claimed by the doctor in billing for his own time is justified by my diagnoses and the tests ordered. The insurance company will also perform various checks for unbundling, which is breaking out and billing for individual services from a service that should be billed as a single comprehensive one. For example, they try to catch cases where a practice might perform a five-view knee X-ray, which is a procedure in its own right, with its own allowable reimbursement, and then bill it as five individual X-rays at a higher total price.

In our fee-for-service system, this game between providers of care and those paying for it is an old one and benefits no one, least of all the patient. For a half century now, the relationship between providers and those who pay for medical care has been like that Whac-A-Mole game you remember from the game rooms of your youth. Medical providers keep popping up new ways to beat the system. Those paying the bills try to quickly whack them down with their mallet, only to have them pop up in a new place in the next instant.

When the insurance company has determined which charges they'll pay, the bill submitted by my doctor is compared to the benefits offered by my insurance, which will likely be different even within that same insurance company from those of another patient with a different employer. They'll determine how much my particular insurance plan should pay for each of these various services. If my insurance plan has deductibles—i.e. if it only pays for services after I have already spent a certain amount—they'll check if I have reached those levels of self-payment. If there are limits on certain services, they'll check to see if I have exceeded them.

If all goes smoothly, the insurance company then sends a check back to the practice. That will arrive together with a statement of which charges it has approved and how much it's paying for each one claimed. The practice then determines what remains to be billed directly to me, it prints a paper bill, mails it to me, and the practice's accounts receivable system is set up to keep track of my bill and the payments that I make. If I don't pay it all at once, there's a monthly statement of my balance.

In the specific case of my annual physical, this entire mechanism has been unleashed for the practice to bill for about $480 of medical services and receive from the insurance company about $240. My doctor works in a practice of thirty-one physicians and eight nurse practitioners, and they employ twenty people just to administer this obsolete system of payment: ten data entry clerks, three billing specialists, three accounts receivable specialists, two patient account specialists, and two precertification nurses.

If, as a result of my physical, my doctor determines that I need some additional medical attention, he might refer me to a physician outside his practice. Now the complexity goes up dramatically. Suppose for a moment that as he examines me he's concerned that I might have some small nodules in my thyroid. These are common and about 10% of people my age have them. Since once in a while they can turn into thyroid cancer, which is not a good thing, they should be checked. To perform this check, my doctor refers me to another physician for an ultrasound imaging of my thyroid.

Even before he makes the referral, his staff needs to check the details of my insurance coverage, as it's likely there are requirements to refer to certain outside practitioners and not to others. That referral may require a pre-authorization—a phone call to the insurance company (or to a company the insurance company has contracted with) to justify the referral. The people on the other end of the telephone earn their keep by making referrals difficult.

Once a doctor that my insurance company will accept is selected and the referral is authorized, I'm sent on my way to get the ultrasound. It will probably take place in a hospital outpatient department, and this entire billing process will occur twice again—first by the hospital whose outpatient department I've used and second by the physician who will view the ultrasound images and interpret them. If that physician determines that a needle biopsy is needed, a pathology group is added to review and interpret the biopsy sample, and possibly a further subspecialist (a cytologist) in yet another group is added to do a final check of the results.

This is not the stuff of television medical dramas. It's a straightforward referral that represents a common and modest step up in complexity from my routine annual physical. This is the day in and day out stuff of medical care. The ultrasound and biopsy are more expensive than my physical, and might cost about $1,500 in addition to my original $480 visit. But to manage the payments for this, the entire insurance reimbursement process—the collection and maintenance of patient and insurance information, the billing, the auditing and analysis by the insurance company, the partial payment to the physician practice, the billing and collection of the balance to the patient—is repeated five times over. It has been separately invoked by my own physician, the hospital whose outpatient department performed the scan, the endocrinologist who interprets the ultrasound, the pathologist who interprets the biopsy, and perhaps the subspecialist cytologist who checks the result.

Should I be unfortunate enough to have a real problem, the billing complexity now escalates exponentially. There will be additional imaging technology such as CT scans, nuclear medicine imaging, and PET (positron emission tomography) scans. Even if they're performed at the same hospital, each of these additional imaging procedures likely brings its own physician group into the cycle for interpretation of the results. My treatment might include the services of an oncologist and a surgeon, and possibly those of a radiation oncologist. Anyone who has experienced a serious illness themselves or with a family member knows how extraordinarily complex and difficult it is to sort through the financial ramifications of such an illness.

No one needs to be reminded that there's a lot of paperwork in dealing with health insurance. The blame is often laid at the feet of insurance companies—they were made the villains in the Affordable Care Act. But the real problem is something else: an inefficient Rube Goldberg system of payment for medical care that still persists in a world that has long since left behind any rationale for doing it this way. The way we treat medical care today—as a vast collection of independent and separately processed little insurance reimbursements—is an anachronism. It's the health care equivalent of what it would be like to have our phone calls (and e-mails and tweets) still going through a switchboard.

A common prescription for cutting through this paperwork jungle is a so-called "single payer" system. In such a system, there is just one insurance company and one set of rules. It helps a little, but not even remotely enough. Medicare is the nation's single-payer health insurance system and its per capita costs have risen over the years faster, not slower, than those of other health care sectors. Most importantly, a single-payer system leaves the real drivers of cost untouched because it preserves the underlying insurance paradigm that's at the heart of the problem. The Blue Hammer thought experiment earlier in this chapter is a single-payer system in the way I described it. Its absurdity lies in the lack of control over what's done and how it's done, and not in the inefficiency of the check writing. Continuing to write checks for too many of the wrong things, but doing it more efficiently, is no solution to anything.

This process of submitting and paying claims is not only inefficient and ignores the underlying drivers of cost, it also misdirects our efforts. Excellent health care is well-coordinated care. Yet the payment mechanism of paying for myriad individual elements of service encourages and locks into our thinking a view of health care as a collection of distinct and relatively independent events. We spend a lot of money on trying to put back into health care the coordination and integration that we have taken out through the workings of how we pay for it.

This insurance paradigm for how we pay for health care is a concept that made perfect sense once, but that has long since outlived its time. It makes health care inefficient and it's at the root of the perverse incentives that damage our health care system. It's a relic of another age and genuine health care reform will only come from moving on to something better.

5

Moving Forward

American health care needs to be set on a new foundation. Too many things are wrong, not from malice or ignorance, but just as the result of the accumulation of structures over the years that have outlived their usefulness. The danger in the Affordable Care Act isn't so much that it does harm, but that it claims to fix things that it only puts duct tape on. When something is visibly broken, at least its repair remains on the to-do list, even if we defer it for a while. But an inadequate repair is often worse than none at all. The problem drops from sight until it breaks again later and it is invariably more expensive to repair than if it had been done right in the first place.

We need a new foundation and I believe there are four cornerstones to it. The biggest cornerstone is quality—our health care should be the best in the world. Its costs should be under control and sensible compared with other priorities in our society. It should be paid for honestly and not with borrowings. It should be universal. The rest of this book is about how we might achieve that.

My thoughts about how to fix health care started with a small epiphany. In 2005, I was invited to speak to an international conference of physicists who were meeting in Tennessee. While that might seem an unlikely venue for a politician, my formal education was in that field, and the novelty of a sitting governor with a degree in physics was sufficient to produce an invitation to speak.

Following my presentation, Dr. Cecilia Jarlskog, a mathematician from Lund University in Sweden, took the podium. She had been a member of the Nobel Prize Committee for Physics, and talked about the way that knowledge in the sciences progresses. Her thesis was that there's a cycle to understanding: we start out solving problems with what she called the "cookbook" approach. We treat problems individually, with recipes to solve them that work, or almost work, or sometimes work, or don't work, but we don't know why. The problems themselves are seen as individual and disconnected. The cookbook grows.

Then something happens and we find a way to look at the problems from a different perspective. We find a new way of looking at the world that reveals an underlying structure we didn't see before. Once in a long while, that new understanding might be the product of an individual genius like an Einstein or a Darwin; the rest of the time it's a gradual process that involves a great many people and lots of blind alleys. But there comes a point when we suddenly realize that if we'll just come around to the side here and look at things from this different angle, we can see what's really going on. We can throw away the cookbook; we can see into things and *understand* why one approach works and another doesn't. We can use the new insight to predict. And then, as time goes on, we find new problems that even this new perspective doesn't illuminate, we start a new cookbook, and the cycle begins again.

She was talking about physics, but as I sat listening it struck me: *This is precisely where health care is today.* We have a problem to solve, let's say the high cost of drugs. Lots of recipes are proposed: buying from Canada, price controls on manufacturers, generic substitution, preferred drug lists, electronic prescribing, negotiating rebates, and hiring companies to call doctors and ask them to change their prescribing habits, to name a few. Some of these recipes help and some don't, but they're all just recipes—stopgaps that have to serve until we gain an understanding of just *why* those drugs are so expensive and fix that problem.

In health care, we've built up a vast cookbook of ways to deal with our problems—with costs, with quality, and with accessibility. We added a lot of pages to the cookbook in the Affordable Care Act. Over the years, some of our recipes have worked, some have helped, some have hurt, and many have been of no consequence at all. Now we've arrived at a place where the cookbook is so large and the recipes so numerous that we've lost our bearings.

The light that went on for me in that auditorium was that rather than continuing to expand the recipe count—which I've done my share of over the years—we should be trying instead to find a fresh approach. We need a new angle from which to view things. We're juggling too many things; we need to unify and simplify our understanding. That's what I'm setting out to do now: to take a fresh look, from a different perspective, and try to solve this problem.

The road ahead

My education isn't traditional for the world of politics. It's in the sciences and people will sometimes ask me, usually as a friendly joke, how I use that in the governor's office. There are areas where it's definitely a weakness. There have been many times where, had I known more about the law, or about history, I could have done a better job. But I've also found that the sciences give you a way of thinking about things that has some real strengths as well. The most useful of these over the years has been to think about problems in terms of multistep solutions—keep in mind where you want to go, but then break the journey down into manageable steps. Find some intermediate places to stop, regroup, and move on to the next step. As a way of thinking, it's very different from the "problem–solution–move on to the next problem" approach that dominates the world of public policy and is very evident in what we've just done with health reform.

I'm very literal in the way I think about things, and this technique of breaking up complicated problems into manageable pieces is no different—I think about problems in terms of crossing a stream. If you're traveling and come to a stream without a bridge, there are a couple of ways to proceed. One strategy is to back up, run hard, let out a yell, leap as far as you can, and hope that you'll land safely on the far bank. Once in a while you make it, but most often, it's a poor strategy that lands you in the water. The other approach is to find some stepping stones and make the crossing one step at a time. I imagine those stepping stones literally: some slippery, some solid; the next step sometimes small, sometimes a leap. It can still be a difficult crossing, but breaking the problem up into discrete steps is a powerful way of approaching it.

That's how I'm approaching health care in the pages ahead. We're going to logically work our way across the stream to a better system, one stepping stone at a time. There will be six of them.

First stepping-stone: Fairness and dignity. This first step is to set for ourselves some ethical principles that will be our framework. This book is about the organization of the delivery and payment for medical care (rather than the rich and separate field of medical and professional ethics). In that context, we're going to establish three principles. First, the system should be universal: that there is an underlying level of medical care that we believe is the right of any American who is breathing. Second, that Americans equally situated should be treated equally, both in terms of how much they pay and what they receive. Third, that every American should be able to access that medical care with dignity and privacy.

Second stepping-stone: Costs. Get to the core of why health care costs so much. This has to get at deeper causes than the usual discussion of new technology, new drugs, high prices, and evident overutilization: these are symptoms. I'm going to establish that the root cause is that we have everywhere in our health care system systematically smothered the economic tension that creates value. Once we accept that as the underlying issue, we have a solid place to stand and can plan our next steps around a path to reestablishing that tension in a practical and ethical way.

Third stepping-stone: A new approach to managing the delivery of health care. I've called this managing hypercomplexity—thinking in a different way about how to shape the workings of our health care system. Health care is so big, has so many independent players, and is so loosely connected that traditional organizational concepts fail. We need new rules. We'll look at two other examples of hypercomplexity—a market economy and evolution—and learn things from how they work that we can apply to health care.

Fourth stepping-stone: Quality. We'll show how to place quality —by which I mean adherence to evidence-based standards with room for professional judgment—in a far more central role than it plays today. This fourth step is a comprehensive approach to establishing standards and auditing the performance of health care delivery against them.

Fifth stepping-stone: Systems of care. In this step, we'll reorganize the delivery of health care around organized systems of care. We'll add a new dimension as well by making those systems, however they choose to organize their internal operations and payments, responsible for the overall quality of care. It will be as if Blue Cross were to be responsible not only for paying your medical bills, but also for the quality of care you receive.

Sixth and final stepping-stone: Paying for health care with a national trust account and vouchers. This last stepping-stone does two things. It allows us to control the resources we put into health care and retreat from an open-ended entitlement. It also empowers individuals to own and control their own health care. We're going to collect the money we need through the tax system and place it in a reserved trust account. Out of that account we'll give each individual

American a voucher with which to purchase their basic health care from whomever they want.

Before I leave this sixth stepping stone, let me acknowledge that its description contains the "tax" word with its ability to promptly suck all the oxygen out of any room. Let me be clear: this is not about adding cost or doing more things; nor is it about expanding government control over health care. It's just the opposite: this is about reducing costs, doing fewer things, managing our deficit, and reversing the continued slide toward greater and greater direct government control over the health care of more and more Americans. If we can summon enough confidence in our government to allow it to be the vehicle for assembling these funds but keep its hands off the details of how they're spent, we can fashion a fairer and more efficient system—a private sector solution. Before leaping to pigeonhole this approach by its use of the tax system, I respectfully ask that you read on with an open mind.

The Aunt Naomi Test

As must be clear from my story of the physics conference in 2005, I've often found ideas that first come into being in the context of science to have something to say in unrelated fields as well. The value of simplicity and clarity is one of them. When I was studying physics in college, I had a professor named Don Edwards. Speaking about physics, he told us that if we were asked a question by a lay person about something in our field and we had to beg off because the questioner didn't have some prerequisite expertise, that was a failure on our part, not the questioner's.

He said, "If you have to say, 'Well, that's a good question, but until you take a course in differential equations, I really can't explain it to you,' then that's just an admission on your part that you don't really have command of the subject. If you did, you could give a respectful and informative response to any interested listener." He added that it's really hard to have that kind of a command of complicated and difficult subjects.

I've found that principle true in many other places, and it's been at the core of my approach to governing. When I have to explain my rationale for a complicated course of action, my version of Professor Edwards' rule is the "Aunt Naomi Test." Naomi Oswalt was my aunt, and she and her husband lived with us for a while, and then next door, when I was growing up. She had a high school education and worked behind the counter at the local soda fountain. Her husband, Ozzie, left school at fourteen. He delivered milk and worked as a bookkeeper for the local Chevy dealership. Naomi was intelligent and interested; she read the newspapers and thought about the things she read, but she certainly wasn't "sophisticated"; I doubt she would have known what a white paper was. She had an enormous amount of common sense though: I especially remember coming back to my rural home as a Harvard student with the latest ideas from Cambridge, and she would listen, and sometimes she'd nod in understanding, but sometimes she'd raise an eyebrow and gently suggest that I might want to think a bit more about that one.

My Aunt Naomi Test is just this: when I think I have an idea about a course of action, I do a thought experiment. I test my own thinking for clarity and command of the subject by imagining explaining it to Aunt Naomi. I have to make that explanation respectfully, without reference to white papers or ideology or the opinions of others. When I do so, even all these years after her death, I can still see in my mind what questions she would ask and what her reaction might be. I can see whether she would agree or whether she would raise that eyebrow and suggest that her educated young nephew perhaps needed to think again. Health reform needs a lot of Aunt Naomi Tests. In every field—in art, in literature, in politics—simplicity and clarity are virtues. Finding the essence, simplifying things, is much harder than making things more complex; much harder but much more rewarding.

Naomi had one guaranteed question. Whenever I fell into complaining what was wrong with something, she would let me go on for a little, and then interrupt and ask, "What would you do?" I've been complaining in these pages for a while about what is wrong with health care and with President Obama's reform. Now Aunt Naomi interrupts and asks her question.

What would I do? Let's begin.

6

Stepping-Stone One:
Dignified, Fair, and Universal

. . . in which we move to our first stepping-stone. We
identify three ethical principles as a starting point:
accessing medical care with dignity and privacy; ensuring
that Americans who are similarly situated are treated
similarly; making basic health care universal and a right
of Americans. We then look at America's successful and
well-liked Social Security system to see what can be
learned from its success to guide us.

Dignity and privacy

In the 1980s I was chief executive of my managed care company, and we operated a health maintenance organization (HMO)
in Pittsburgh. Our customers were employer-based—private companies, unions, and public sector employees—and we had no involvement with public sector health programs such as Medicaid or
Medicare. This was not any philosophical or business decision on
our part, but simply that those public sector programs at that time
had few ways for the private sector to participate.

Our HMO was successful and well-regarded in the Pittsburgh community, and we were approached at one point by the Pennsylvania

Department of Public Welfare. They asked if we would contract with them for Medicaid patients, using the same benefit package we offered to others; they were trying to bring their Medicaid program more into the mainstream of health care there. We wanted to be cooperative and agreed to contract with them, but I remember offering the opinion that we would find few takers, as the existing Medicaid benefit package was more generous in several ways than our private sector offering. A rational person who qualified for Medicaid should prefer the benefits of that system. The months after we began enrollment proved me wrong and it turned out that we signed up a substantial number of Medicaid beneficiaries.

I wanted to understand why, and on a visit to one of our primary care centers in Pittsburgh we identified a woman with a child who had come to us through the Pennsylvania Medicaid program. I approached her politely, identified myself, and asked her, "Why?" She had a simple and straightforward answer: she took out her identification card, held it up for me to see, and said, "Because now my card looks just like everyone else's, and my son and I don't get treated like second-class people." It stopped me cold. I'd become so involved as a young executive in the mechanics of operating a health care system that I'd forgotten her basic and completely understandable human need to be able see her doctor with dignity and privacy. A young woman and her son on Medicaid, names long since lost, thankfully brought me back to earth. As I watched the recent health reforms unfold, I wished that all those policy experts with their spreadsheets could have been there with me.

The founding principles of our nation are drawn from a deep well: a strongly held and historical belief in the natural rights and dignity of our citizens. The founding document of our nation declares that all men are created equal. It asserts that we're endowed by our Creator with inalienable rights. Nowhere does it mention that the path to those rights passes through a definition of "percent of poverty" or the actions of any department of human services.

Before Thomas Jefferson wrote the Declaration of Independence, he wrote that, "A free people [claim] their rights as derived from the laws of nature, and not as the gift of their chief magistrate."

I doubt that our nation's Founders had any premonition of how important our various forms of social insurance would become, but the ability to access basic medical care has now—very properly—become a de facto right in America. As we work to figure out how to guarantee that right, I believe those Founders would pray that our starting point would be, once again, the dignity of our citizens, not simple political calculation, and especially not styled as a gift from latter-day magistrates, this time installed in Washington.

Modern society continues to grow more mobile and our place in it more anonymous and disconnected from traditional relationships. We all need a helping hand from time to time, but the structures of family and neighbors that have held out those hands are growing rarer with each passing year. This is a role that we're more and more assuming as a society—mostly through government, but also through our nonprofit and faith-based institutions.

My mother, brother, and I grew up in my grandmother's home. We lived in a village of eleven hundred people, and my grandmother had ten children who grew to adulthood. During most of my younger years, nine of those ten children and their families lived in or around that village. There was an automatic support system for her when she needed it. When her children had some need they called on their siblings' families. In one generation it all changed: the next generation —mine—is scattered around the country. There are far fewer ties of family to backstop us if we get into difficulty. Those aunts and uncles of mine worked in factories, delivered mail, and served food in the school cafeteria. They weren't wealthy, but I remember that world clearly, and I remember how important it was for them to face the world with dignity and independence. The woman and her son who belonged to the Pennsylvania Medicaid program didn't teach me a lesson, she reminded me of something I already knew.

In my adult lifetime, we've vastly expanded the scope of our helping hands, but the way in which we've done it troubles me a lot. We've become very technocratic and financial in the way we look at these responsibilities and forget the need for dignity and privacy that those we're helping must feel. We can do a lot of damage with our approach. We firmly embed in the minds of some of our children at an early age that they are part of a separate group of poorer citizens who are designated "free and reduced lunch" or "at risk." Right at the time when these children are most impressionable and when they're forming lifelong self-images, we remind them repeatedly in school that they're different. We're doing the same with health care, and our recent reform has exacerbated it. Perhaps a person who has worked and earned health benefits for her family for years finds herself unemployed. Are we really going to tell her, "If you want help with medical care, just go down to the welfare office and sign up. Bring lots of personal information and stand in line with the unmarried pregnant teenager."

This is not just some conservative small town objection on my part. In Tennessee, we have a health insurance program for children called "Cover TN." This is our implementation of the federal Children's Health Insurance Program, known by its acronym, CHIP. It offers free or very low cost comprehensive health insurance to children who live in families whose incomes are above the levels at which they would qualify for Medicaid. In Tennessee, we offer free insurance to children in families with incomes of less than about $55,000 for a family of four. These families are some of the same ones that the Affordable Care Act has now included in its Medicaid expansions and the subsidized plans of the Exchange.

One of the challenges we face is getting parents to enroll children who are eligible. Firmly middle-class parents—urban and rural both—who have never been to a Human Services office will come to one of our sign-up sessions at a shopping center or at their church. This is something they want for their child. We're required by law to evaluate them first for Medicaid, but when we begin that process, there are always some who just won't do it; they're not willing to engage in that way with the welfare system. They walk away.

I have a visceral dislike of where we have come to: a new class of "magistrates" dispensing health care and reduced-price lunches and a dozen other things to millions of supplicants, some of whom need genuine charity, but most of whom are ordinary, proud Americans who need some help. There is a larger picture here than efficiently dispensing charity. We should eliminate "percentage of poverty" permanently from our lexicon and national discussions, and health care is a good place to start. Sixty years ago, Harry Truman wanted a health care system that treated every American on an equal footing. It's hard to believe that sixty years later we would have *retreated* from that goal.

Alice and Bob: different employers

Our second principle addresses some inequities that already pervade health care and which our recent reforms have made worse. We all know that expanding health care coverage means moving a lot of money around. Health care is expensive, and if you have diabetes or heart disease or cancer, your treatment costs the same whether your income is $10,000 or $100,000. Some people are going to need subsidies. However, there are great inequities in how that subsidy is distributed. Two Americans that a reasonable person might think deserved to be treated comparably are often actually treated very differently.

Let's do a thought experiment: It's after the year 2014, and the Affordable Care Act health care reforms are in place. Alice is a widow with three children and an income of $40,000. She works for a large company—let's say a bank—that offers health insurance, which she takes. She doesn't love her job, it's just okay, but the benefits are important to her.

Bob is a single parent with three children as well, makes the same $40,000 and works for a small building contractor that's owned by a friend of his. He loves his job and the fellows he works with. His employer doesn't offer insurance and is small enough to be exempt from the mandate to do so. Bob hasn't had health insurance for several years, but now is able to buy it through the Exchange. His health insurance costs about $14,200 annually. He pays about $2,000 and the subsidy from the taxpayers is over $12,000. He is very satisfied with the arrangement.

Alice looks at this, and says, "Wait a minute. I've made compromises and tough choices to make sure I have good health insurance for me and my family. Even my share of my health insurance premiums is much larger than Bob's, and in a real sense I'm paying my employer's share of those premiums as well. If he weren't paying for health benefits, he could pay me more—thousands of dollars more—and that would really help us. Tell me exactly why I should make these compromises and sacrifices to be responsible—to make sure that I've provided for me and my children—and *then* have to stand and watch while my tax dollars go to pay most of Bob's insurance, who's made none of these hard choices? We both make $40,000, our families are alike, yet he gets more than $12,000 of help from the taxpayers every year and I get nothing."

This comparison of Bob and Alice is not an issue of the wealthier objecting to contributing to those with less income; in health care, that's a given. It's just the issue of the very different treatment of two people who are in similar situations. In the way we've placed heavily subsidized insurance alongside employer-paid insurance, we've created deep inequities in the different way that two people in equivalent circumstances are treated.

Alice and Bob: different cities

There are other inequities in the way that people who are similarly situated are treated in our health care system as well. The

Dartmouth Atlas Project has documented for more than twenty years the large disparities—sometimes greater than 2:1—in the cost of health care in different regions of the United States. This was discussed extensively during the health reform debates leading up to the Affordable Care Act. That project has looked into the reasons for these differences, and other researchers have taken their data and done the same. The results are clear: these regional differences are not urban-rural variations and they are not simply explained by differences in the health status or income of people living there. Especially, they're not explained by differences in the quality of care in the region: the quality was frequently found to be superior in the lower-cost parts of the country. (Their data, by the way, is now suddenly undergoing intense scrutiny because of the influence it had on President Obama's health reform. I feel certain that some contrary points will be made—that's the strength of scientific research—but there is a lot of solid underlying truth in what they've done.

What these regional variations do reflect is simply discretionary decisions made by local physicians. In those parts of the country with higher costs, patients had more things done to them, or they were charged more, or both. But the *quality* of the medical care they received was often unrelated to how much they were paying for it. This comes as no surprise to any of us who have worked in health care in different parts of the country.

While this regional variation is usually discussed in the context of lowering health care costs, it has another dimension, as well, in the issues of fairness and equal treatment. Let's revisit Alice and Bob, but this time they live in different cities. Alice lives in Minneapolis and Bob in Dallas. They're both paying Medicare premiums through a payroll deduction: 1.45% themselves and another 1.45% from their employers. The Medicare hospital trust fund is already spending more than it is taking in, and will be out of money before long. Bob and Alice will each likely have to absorb an increase in Medicare taxes in the near future (or see the diversion to Medicare of other funds that could have benefited them in other ways).

Both Minneapolis and Dallas are modern, middle American cities and they have nearly identical cost-of-living indexes. But the average Medicare spending for health care for those on Medicare in Minneapolis is $6,700; the average in Dallas is $10,100—a full 50% higher, half again as much. Furthermore, in Dallas, the annual rate of growth is higher as well. That cost disparity is going to get worse, not better.

Alice might reasonably ask: "In Minneapolis, we have excellent health care at a reasonable cost. Just why should I have to absorb a tax increase to support a more wasteful system in Dallas? If the expensive parts of the country had their costs under control like we do, the Medicare trust fund wouldn't be going bankrupt nearly as fast. Don't raise *my* taxes; Bob, tell Dallas to get its act together."

Our principle of people similarly situated being treated similarly extends to geography as well as employers. We don't allow these kinds of disparities to take place in our Social Security payments and we should object to their existence in health care as well.

Alice and Bob: paying more and getting less

Let's visit Alice and Bob again. Alice still works at that bank, and her children are covered under her employer's health insurance plan. They don't qualify for any of the public programs to provide insurance to children because Alice has access to insurance at her workplace. Bob is still at the small contractor, and while he doesn't have insurance right now, his children do. The children comfortably qualify for the CHIP program in their state and have free comprehensive insurance.

Alice has grown to accept some of the disparity in how she and Bob are treated. She's of a generous mind, is happy to have her job with benefits, and doesn't begrudge Bob's children getting insurance through another route, even a heavily subsidized one. But now she takes a look at just what that insurance covers, and finds that Bob's children have a better deal. She pays $25 for a prescription for one of her children; Bob pays $5. Her children's plan doesn't cover dental services; Bob's children have that coverage. Without being selfish, Alice might well say: "I don't mind Bob's kids having federally funded insurance; kids need it and I'm glad that Bob's children have it just as my own do. But Bob's son having *better* insurance than my daughter, why should that be?"

Several years ago, I had to make substantial cuts in Tennessee's Medicaid program—TennCare. We didn't cut children from the program or reduce their benefits, but we did for many adults. A political problem that had deeply undermined public support for TennCare was one of perception. There were a lot of ordinary Tennesseans who were working hard and earning their health care benefits. These same Tennesseans were starting to become aware that their neighbors who were receiving benefits through TennCare were not only paying a lot less but also getting a lot more. Very few begrudged someone health insurance or even the public subsidy that made it possible, but they did resent the fact that TennCare was not only cheaper, it was more comprehensive. It was an accurate perception. Someone who belonged to TennCare through one of its extra categories—those who were in the "uninsured" or "uninsurable" categories—had a noticeably better benefit package than many with employer-based plans. Often the coverage was dramatically better than that of small business owners or individuals who were purchasing their own coverage.

This disparity is about to become even more widespread and visible with the Affordable Care Act. There will be many more Americans in the very Comprehensive Medicaid Program, and in the subsidized programs offered through Exchanges, it will be attractive for many people to purchase quite comprehensive insurance plans. That will lead in turn to a TennCare-like situation where those receiving a subsidy will have more comprehensive benefits than their counterparts paying their own way in employer-based plans. I learned during our TennCare reforms that most people were generous; they thought it a moral obligation to make sure that others had access to health care. On the whole, they didn't object to the coverage being the same as theirs. They definitely, however, did *not* see it as a moral responsibility to ensure that others had more comprehensive coverage than they themselves did. Instead, they were offended by it. If Alice is a little upset with the additional benefits that Bob's children have, think how she's going to feel when she figures out that she works hard for her family's silver plan, and the guys who can't hold a job and hang out all day at the pool hall have the platinum one.

Our second principle of fairness is straightforward. We need to return our health care system to a more equitable state, where people in equivalent situations are treated the same. This is an ethical matter, but it's also a political one. It will be difficult to maintain political support for any system that is regarded as unfair by a broad swath of average Americans.

Alice and Bob: lifestyle

There's a final and related fairness issue in the way in which our health care system handles lifestyle choices. Smoking and obesity are habits that arise from personal choices and affect the cost of health care. It would certainly seem fair to recognize this in the way in which we pay for health care—perhaps those with such habits should pay more to reflect their higher health care costs. I want to offer a view that's contrary to the conventional wisdom (and my own actions in the past) on this.

A significant and growing amount of disease in America is not the result of infectious agents or unpredictable failings of our bodies. Instead, it's self-induced. Smokers experience health problems resulting from their habit, including a variety of cancers, heart disease, and lung disease. The additional annual health care costs of a smoker vary by age and other factors but are typically 20–30% more than those of a nonsmoker. Those who are obese and who fail to exercise likewise experience chronic health problems including Type 2 diabetes and heart disease. Their annual medical costs are typically a third more than those of a person of normal weight. Should a nonsmoker have to pay higher premiums themselves to cover the extra costs of medical care for someone who smokes two packs a day? Should someone who exercises and keeps their weight under control have to pay for someone who doesn't?

There have been attempts to address this by, in some fashion, increasing the relative costs of insurance for smokers or for someone whose weight qualifies them as "obese," the latter usually defined as someone with a body mass index (BMI) over 30. (This would equate to a five foot eleven inch man with a weight of over 215 pounds). The Affordable Care Act specifically anticipates charging additional premiums for smokers (but not for those who are overweight). I've recently done just that with a public health care program in Tennessee. In our subsidized small-business health insurance program, we effectively charge additional premiums for both smokers and those who are substantially overweight. This has an aura of fairness about it: people need to take responsibility for their lifestyle choices. There's another side to this coin however. Smoking and obesity are personal choices that are the current and well-deserved targets of critics. They have a real impact on the overall cost of health care. But they're hardly the only risky behavior that people engage in.

Let's visit Alice and Bob one last time. This time, they work for the same employer. Alice smokes cigarettes and her employer charges her more for her health care in compensation. Bob doesn't smoke and pays a lower rate. Alice has a complaint, and it's a legitimate one: "I smoke, and I understand why I should pay more. But why not Bob, who drinks too much and eats red meat seven days a week? Why not Carol, who scuba dives and rock climbs? Why not Dave, who rides a big motorcycle?"

What Alice is pointing out is that once we start taking the various health risks of different lifestyles into account, we step onto a slippery slope. There's no fairness in punishing one lifestyle choice for its health risks while ignoring another choice that may be even worse ("You shouldn't smoke, but it's okay to be a heavy drinker"). Yet we'd create an unmanageable monster if we tried to continuously fine tune a person's cost of health care to reflect their participation in risky behavior. Even were we to attempt it, any penalties or rate differentials we might set up in response to these risky behaviors become meaningless when we try to impose them on those with lower incomes. For example, imagine a person enrolled in the essentially free Medicaid system because he can't pay for health care. Once the Affordable Care Act becomes effective, that category alone will encompass one in every four Americans. For that group, we can impose all the penalties or extra premiums we want, but they can't pay them and we're not going to deny them health coverage for that reason.

We also open an emotional debate (and invite the courts into it) as to just where personal responsibility begins and ends. My own personal view regards obesity as a failure of personal responsibility —the lack of enough self-discipline to push back from the table. But there are others who very legitimately argue that it has a genetic component, or a glandular one, or even a psychological basis that should be regarded as a behavioral disability. We've discussed earlier the way in which we've been steadily moving a range of behavioral issues from the world of morality to the world of medicine. Anyone with a friend who smokes cigarettes knows how truly addictive the habit is—where do we draw the line between what's a matter of personal responsibility and what's a medical or behavioral problem in its own right?

(Alice could also make another, more ghoulish, point: her lifetime costs as a smoker may well be *less* than Bob's because the extra annual cost from her smoking habit while she's alive could be more than offset by the fact that she is likely to die a decade sooner. Perhaps she should have a premium *decrease*.)

Personal responsibility is an important value in our own lives and in our democracy. I've tried over the years in the public arena to incorporate it into the way we look at areas like education and health care. But with health care, I've found it very difficult to incorporate that value in how we pay for care in any practical or fair way. Most Americans would agree that preexisting conditions shouldn't be a barrier to obtaining health insurance; we've just placed that concept firmly into law. Opening the doors to health insurance for those who have existing health problems has been a central goal of reform efforts for a long time. Yet a great many pre-existing conditions have their roots in lifestyle choices. If we value in our society—as we obviously do—the notion that access to health care should be independent of preexisting conditions, the logical follow-on is to make it also independent of lifestyle choices.

We all have different genes and different behaviors, we've all made different choices in the past, both good and bad, and we live our lives in different ways. Risky behavior and a failure to assume responsibility for our own health has far deeper consequences than just the size of our health insurance premiums—they are major determinants of the quality and length of our lives. Educating us about the consequences of different behaviors and even offering assistance with altering them should be a central part of our vision for the role of public health. But when it comes to direct medical care, the sensible course seems to be to simply say: "Lead your life as you see fit. If you need medical care, it may just be the luck of the draw or you may have helped it along with the way you eat or what you do in your spare time—it's hard to tell. But that's water over the dam. In the here and now, you need medical care, and in America it will be there for you."

Universal coverage

There are a lot of ways in which we might decide to organize and pay for health care, but we've reached a time in America when we need to go ahead and take the step of making it universal. Earlier in this chapter we explored the idea that there is at least a base level of health care that has become, for all practical purposes, a right of Americans. If we accept that to be the case, the next step is to assume the obligation and go ahead and ensure that right for everyone. That's a statement of values, of course, but also one of practicality. We've moved ever closer over the years to achieving complete coverage, but even with the Affordable Care Act, there will still be about twenty-three million uninsured people in our country—one in every thirteen. We're not going to let them suffer or die for lack of medical care and so that means we still need to maintain a messy system to indirectly subsidize care for them. With the Affordable Care Act, we'll also need an extensive bureaucratic apparatus to enforce mandates, assign fines, and process what will likely be millions of exceptions. Even setting aside the moral issue, there's a practical one. We're 93% of the way there. Taking the final step and creating a uniform, universal system sweeps away in an instant a great deal of the complexity and cost in our health care system.

The Social Security model

This first stepping-stone of ours has been to establish some underlying principles to guide our thinking. I've suggested some: the dignity of abandoning the paternalism of a visibly means-tested system; the inherent fairness of treating citizens in comparable situations the same; neutrality when it comes to personal lifestyles; universal care. As you've followed this, you may have agreed or disagreed with individual items. I've discussed these ideas with others in the past, and your reaction might be a common one I've experienced: "I agree with what you've said in theory but it's just too different from what we have now to be practical. Interesting, but unrealistic."

But that's not right. When our nation first began assuming a role in providing social insurance, we set up an institution embodying these principles almost exactly—Social Security. That institution has grown and prospered for three-quarters of a century now. It may well be the most popular government program of all time. The reason it has been so popular and stable is precisely *because* it's firmly grounded in a sense of dignity and fairness, and not because of the technical workings of the program. Its support is far broader than those programs in the social arena that are means tested. Politicians tinker with it at their peril, as President George W. Bush discovered in 2005.

To start with, Social Security has an inherent dignity about it. It doesn't appear to citizens as some government largesse or welfare payment to benefit them in old age. Instead, it reads as a trust in which they've invested through the payroll taxes they've paid over the years. The right to those benefits is something they own. When the time comes for each of us to start withdrawing our "invest-ment" in that trust, we simply receive a check that we then use as we please. We get back the money we have paid in, it's not "redistrib-uted" to someone else. (There is actually some redistribution going on, but it's modest and silent.) When we purchase something at the store with the money we receive, there's no signal to anyone about our economic status; the store clerk doesn't know if we're spending our last dollar or if we have a million more of them at home.

Social Security completely solves all of the Bob and Alice prob-lems. It solves the equal treatment problem: payment into the sys-tem is based solely on income. Every person who earns $40,000 pays the same amount. There are no complicated arrangements of protected employers or exceptions or subsidies to some employers.

If, as an employer, you pay someone wages, you owe Social Security taxes on those wages. If, as an employee, you receive wages, you pay taxes on those wages. If you're not receiving wages, you don't have to pay.

Likewise, it solves the geographical fairness problem. A person's Social Security check doesn't depend on where he lives, but solely on how much he's earned and contributed over the years. Of course, if someone has worked and retired in a high-cost-of-living part of our country, that will likely have been reflected in how much they've been paid over the years and therefore in higher Social Security benefits. The same principle applies to low-cost-of-living areas as well. That natural effect is the only note that's taken of these regional differences. Social Security doesn't move money from Minneapolis to Dallas like the health care system does.

There's no problem with a disparity of benefits; Social Security rules are the same for everyone. It's blind to lifestyle choices. We don't give smokers a discount on their Social Security taxes because we're reasonably sure they won't live long enough to collect their share of benefits. While it wasn't universal—by far—at its inception, for all practical purposes it has become so.

I should acknowledge at this point that there are well-reported problems with Social Security today, and it's thought that the trust fund will be unable to guarantee the full payments promised in a couple more decades. But this is a completely fake problem. Social Security is a simple trust fund system and the only problem is that Congress has failed in its fiduciary duty as a trustee. Anyone who has done well in an actuarial class in college can tell us exactly how to fix Social Security. There are only two levers, and both of them are manipulated with a simple stroke of the pen—there's no management required here. Congress can alter the taxes being collected so that they are sufficient to pay the checks being written. Or it can alter the size and timing of the checks being written to fit the amount the trust fund is collecting. Or a combination of both.

The problem doesn't lie with Social Security, but with Congress, generous as usual with benefits but unwilling as usual to present the taxpayers an honest bill.

Social Security has other features that are worth observing, as well, as we consider our health care system. While the payments into Social Security take place through the employment system, the program and its trust fund are completely separate from any employer. Social Security is portable in the way we want health care to be. Every citizen owns her own Social Security account. It travels with them throughout their life and the contributions to it and payments from it aren't dependent on the generosity or solvency of any employer or union.

The design of Social Security as a trust fund is an important feature. It's a vital part of the ethos of Social Security—a citizen's ownership of an asset rather than dependence on governmental largess. It's also a good way to keep everyone focused on the accounting. With Social Security, specific tax revenues are paid into a trust fund and the benefits are paid out of it. This is in contrast to an approach of comingling its revenues and expenses with those of general government. We're beginning to dilute that critical feature with the way we do consolidated accounting in the federal government, but it is still essentially a correct description of the program.

Social Security depends on a generational transfer, so there is no financial account that a citizen builds up and then draws from as she might from a funded pension plan. Technically, the asset she acquires as a result of her payments into the trust fund isn't stocks and bonds, but a contract to allow her payments to be used for someone elderly, right now, in exchange for her right later in life to draw from the contributions made by the next generation.

A trust fund design helps to ensure clarity and accountability in the collection of taxes that were imposed for a specific purpose, and the actuarial well-being of the fund can be easily determined. The same concept has been used in other areas where specific taxes and their corresponding expenditures are kept technically separate from general government. Federal unemployment insurance is set up in this fashion, as is the federal Highway Trust Fund. Congress at times has also provided direct appropriations to these trust funds from general government revenues, most recently through the American Recovery and Reinvestment Act of 2009.

As we'll see later, I believe that trust funds have a vital role to play in the future of our health care system. They're already used as the vehicle for providing health insurance by many private employers and state and local governments. The trust fund concept is also used for one component of the federal health care system, the Medicare hospital payment system (Medicare Part A). Trust funds are no magic solution and many of them have been set up but then not properly funded, including as I've just noted, Social Security itself. But they have the potential, if managed responsibly, to bring discipline to the process of setting benefits and coverage. The use of trust funds in a national health care system still leaves open the possibility of additional contributions from specific appropriations. There will always be unforeseen circumstances—the HIV epidemic or a flu pandemic, for example—that might call for such external intervention.

Analogies only go so far, and there are, of course, real differences between how Social Security functions and how we'll have to deal with health care over the years. The big one is that Social Security tailors its benefit—a Social Security check—to the amount paid in over the years, whereas that's impossible to do with health care benefits. Whether someone has an income of $40,000 or $140,000, their basic health insurance costs the same. But when America has already invented a form of social insurance that has been working smoothly for three-quarters of a century and proven immensely popular in addition, we should learn all we can from it.

One thing we should learn is what Social Security teaches us about taxes. Americans generally dislike taxes—as an elected official I can confirm this. But the history of Social Security helps us to observe that lumping everything paid to a government together in one pile and calling it "taxes" obscures what's actually going on. There are taxes and there are taxes. In a broad way, the acceptability of any tax is directly related to the extent to which a taxpayer feels that it's committed to some use that benefits him. Social Security is a perfect example of this. For most Americans, their Social Security taxes are considerably larger than their federal income taxes. However, there are no rallies to cut them because they're directly tied to a desirable benefit to the person who pays them. There are other examples: a gallon of gasoline has substantial federal and state taxes imposed on it, but they're committed to a specific purpose—building roads and bridges—and drivers see the benefit of building those things. There's no gas tax protest movement of any substance. I have friends who are avid supporters of small government and the Tea Party movement, but are perfectly content with paying their Social Security taxes and receiving the benefit.

The taxes that create resentment and opposition are those in which the taxpayer doesn't see the benefit, or worse yet, sees the benefit going elsewhere. Americans recognize some of the need for general taxation; almost all of us recognize the need for a strong military or a diplomatic corps. But when taxes become something being taken from you and me and distributed to others in ways we don't see as benefiting us, we resist. One of the reasons that the Affordable Care Act has encountered so much grass roots opposition is how openly it does just that.

There's no lack of generosity of spirit in America, in fact, quite the opposite. Americans have, time and again, stepped up when the need has arisen. But that generosity is intimately linked to advancing American values. One of those is a belief that when we pay taxes we want to see where they go and we want to be comfortable that they are accomplishing things that we see as beneficial to

7

Stepping-Stone Two:
Why Health Care Is so Expensive

. . . in which we take a realistic look at where American
health care stands in comparison with other nations. We
demonstrate just how much money we actually spend and
the impact it has on our solvency as a nation. Then we
look closely at the cause for this—the systematic
disengagement of the economic tension that creates value
and moderates cost. Having isolated the core problem,
we set out to find the solution.

Not long ago, I had the occasion to visit someone at the Vanderbilt University Medical Center in Nashville. I took the elevator
to the ninth floor and when I stepped off it and started toward the
nursing station, I was suddenly in the midst of the workings of
one of America's great medical centers. This hospital complex, like
its brethren around the nation, is a monument to the vast health
care investment our nation has made in science, in technology, and
in human expertise. Vanderbilt is a sprawling, first-rate American university with many areas of excellence, including a strong
undergraduate school, respected graduate schools of education and
business, and a prominent law school. Its medical center, however,

dominates the university and that dominance makes clear the vastness of the resources that we assign to health care. In the entire university complex, three out of every four employees work at the medical center.

I had to wait a few minutes and walked down the corridor and over to the east windows, where I could look out on Nashville's Edgehill neighborhood. In the summer, Edgehill looks green and peaceful from the ninth floor, but on the ground this is one of our nation's poor inner-city neighborhoods and its health statistics are awful. To find a country to match some of Edgehill's measures of health—the prevalence of low-birth-weight babies, for example—you have to go down the list of country health statistics to places like Albania or Sri Lanka. It would be gratifying if the problem were simply one of having health insurance, but it's not. Nearly all those mothers having the low-birth-weight babies already have comprehensive and generous health insurance through Medicaid. Something else is wrong.

I'm hardly the first person to remark on the incongruity of the wealthy, modern medical center overlooking a poor and unhealthy neighborhood. But let's now walk over to the other side of the building, to the west windows. Here we look out on a landscape that's not poor, but rather a microcosm of America. Nearby, the rooftops identify the homes of comfortable professionals and a little farther away are a collection of both middle- and working-class neighborhoods.

This view doesn't have the easy comparisons of the Edgehill view out the east window, but in many ways it's an even more instructive place to stand. The western view displays just how rich and successful we are as a nation. The neighborhoods lying to the west compare well with the rest of the world in almost every major economic indicator. With one big exception: health care. In that realm, what we have is far more expensive than in other industrialized countries and the results we get are mediocre at best. Those typical Americans out the west window pay almost twice what their peers in other nations do and yet have higher infant mortality, shorter life spans, and more chronic disease.

How did we come to this place over the years? In a nation with a flexible and muscular economy that is so successful in other ways, why is our health care system not world-leading in value and effectiveness as well? Its excess cost and underperformance shortchanges our citizens, undermines our competitiveness, and represents a life-threatening problem to the finances of our nation. Any approach to health reform that doesn't squarely face this issue fails before it begins.

Just how expensive *is* our health care?

Whether we're politicians, business leaders, or regular citizens, we all know that health care in America is expensive. Everyone has an anecdote to relate or a statistic to quote. There are entire books written about the costs of American health care that offer various examples of overutilization and inefficiency. We don't lack data; we're swamped in it. Let's look again for the big shapes.

To begin, we'll put our health care in the context of care in other countries that we might see as useful comparisons to our own. A good way to approach this is to look at the countries that are members of the OECD (Organisation for Economic Co-operation and Development). The OECD today has thirty full members; these are the highly developed countries with advanced market economies. The organization is a premier statistical agency, and has kept and published databases of information about its member countries for decades.

The broadest measure of what we spend on health care in comparison to others is the often-quoted statistic of the percentage of GDP (Gross Domestic Product) that is spent on health care. We should also compare the actual expenditures per capita as well, and Table 3 shows such a set of comparisons for the United States and six of the OECD countries that would commonly be seen as close peers of ours.

Table 3
Comparison of health care costs in seven OECD countries

OECD Member	Health care as a % of GDP		Per capita cost
	1970	2008	2007
Australia	n/a	8.5*	3,501*
Canada	6.9	10.4	4,079
France	5.4	11.2	3,696
Germany	6.0	10.5	3,737
Sweden	6.8	9.4	3,470
United Kingdom	4.5	8.7	3,129
United States	7.1	16.0	7,538

Source: OECDHealthData_FrequentlyRequestedData.xls at www.OECD.org

*Extrapolated

The GDP percentage numbers for 2008 represent the comparisons we all normally hear quoted. The United States expenditures for health care total 16% of our GDP and the next highest among OECD members is France at 11.2%. In the entire OECD list of thirty countries, not just these seven, France is still the next highest. There are no countries between 11% of GDP and our 16%. These GDP comparisons are commonplace, but the per capita costs are even more striking to me. There's a pattern here; these peer countries are all wealthy, highly developed countries with excellent health systems, and they all spend in the rough neighborhood of $3,500 per capita. We stand alone at over twice that expenditure.

There is an encouraging note in these numbers. Note just how recently this disparity has arisen. In 1970, we already dedicated the highest proportion of our GDP to health care, but only by a slight margin. Our health care numbers were very comparable to those of Canada and Sweden (7.1% for the United States versus 6.9% and 6.8% for them). In fact, going back just a bit further to 1960, Canada's GDP percentages were higher than ours. Health care has been an important priority in America for a long time, but the large disparity in cost is a relatively recent phenomenon: most of the problem has arisen only since 1970.

Is health care expensive because it's so good?

Faced with numbers such as these, a common reaction is to say, "Yes, I know it's expensive, but that's because it's so good. America has the best health care in the world." That's plausible, and we can check it against these OECD statistics. One comparison that's often made is the infant mortality rates in these countries. Almost as many people know that we do poorly there as know about GDP percentage comparisons.

Our performance is worth highlighting though, as the ability to bring babies safely into the world integrates many different aspects of a health care system into a simple measurement. The likelihood of a healthy baby depends on many things. Some of them, such as poverty, are realistically beyond the purview of medical care. But many of the factors do relate directly to health care. Access to medical care and advice, competent professionals, and intervention with sophisticated technology when it's needed are all important. The differences in infant mortality rates among nations otherwise similar does tell us something about our health care system. Whether it's yesterday's care given by a doctor traveling on horseback to deliver a baby, or today's care in a modern obstetric practice, producing living, healthy babies is one of the things medical care is supposed to do right.

You already know a part of the answer: that infant mortality rates in modern America are not good. However, as in most things, the trend is even more important. Let's look at the OECD data.

In 1970, we were in the middle of the pack when it came to infant mortality. There were fifteen OECD countries with worse rates than the United States (Austria, Belgium, Czech Republic, Germany, Greece, Hungary, Italy, Korea, Luxembourg, Mexico, Poland, Portugal, Slovak Republic, Spain, and Turkey).

By 1980, we'd fallen a few places so that there were only eleven countries with worse infant mortality rates than us.

By 1990, we'd fallen even further down the list so that we were ahead of only seven (Czech Republic, Hungary, Mexico, Poland, Portugal, Slovak Republic, Turkey).

And by 2006, there were only two OECD countries left with worse infant mortality: Mexico and Turkey. We should thank our stars for Mexico and Turkey; they still have far enough to go that we should be able to hang on to our twenty-eighth place standing (out of thirty) for at least another decade.

When these statistics are pointed out, as has happened often, a common response is to try to explain them away: "Yes, I know they're bad, but America is a big, diverse society. We know we have some problems in our inner cities and on our reservations. But it's unrealistic to compare us with a more homogeneous society; that's not a legitimate test."

Fair enough. So we'll remove entirely from America's statistics all African-American, American Indian, Asian, and Hispanic babies. We're left with only white, non-Hispanic Americans, and the infant mortality numbers are indeed a little better, 5.6 per 1000 instead of 6.7. That means that in 2006, rather than only two countries with worse infant mortality statistics than ours, there were five. We would move up three places, passing Hungary, Poland, and the Slovak Republic into twenty-fifth place.

Think about that for a moment: here's a fundamental measure of the success of our health care system—the ability to assemble our knowledge and technology to bring children safely into this world. Even if you give us the advantage of removing every ethnic group that you think might drag our numbers down, we still rank right near the bottom of the pack.

There's another explanation I sometimes hear: "Okay, I'll agree there's a problem with infant mortality. We may have our priorities wrong, but that's not what our health care system is optimized for.

But, if you have cancer or a stroke or a heart attack, if you're really sick, America is the place to be."

The picture is better here (as it well ought to be with our emphasis on heroic intervention) but still very mixed. We're very average, not exceptional. For breast cancer, we're the best, for colorectal cancer, very near the top. Our laudable emphasis on early detection likely helps these statistics. But we have lots of heart attacks and strokes in America. Our heart attack and ischemic stroke fatality rates are just average. For hemorrhagic strokes, if you're unfortunate enough to have one at all, you'll want to have it elsewhere. We're right near the bottom.

Living long healthy lives

There are a large number of comparisons that can be made among the OECD countries for medical performance with various diseases. Perhaps there's a way to avoid getting bogged down and confused with statistics on a long litany of diseases. Life-threatening conditions such as cancer, heart attacks, and strokes become much more common as we age. Let's look simply at the life expectancy of a sixty-five-year-old and how it compares in different countries. A person has arrived at age sixty-five and now faces the growing prospect of cancer, diabetes, heart disease, and a long list of other complex diseases. This is the stuff we're supposed to be really good at fixing with our specialists and technology. Life expectancy is a simple and indisputable measure (either you're alive or you're not) that integrates a host of much more difficult comparisons.

Here's a striking fact: in the United States, in 1970, the life expectancy of a sixty-five-year-old woman was seventeen years, and that was the *very best* of any OECD country. Not too long ago, we were number one.

By the year 2006, that sixty-five-year-old woman's life expectancy had increased to 20.3 years, which is even better. But the life expectancy in other countries had improved so much more than ours that we were not only knocked out of first place, we'd fallen to number sixteen, in the lower half of the countries we're using for comparisons. (Men occupied twelfth place in 2006, slightly above the median, having fallen from seventh place in 1970.)

This brief discussion of country comparisons certainly doesn't represent a comprehensive academic study on the cost and quality of medical care around the world. But it does help us to cut through the clutter. We've taken a comprehensive and well-respected international database that goes back a long way and looked at it to see if there are any common-sense conclusions that we can draw. There are.

First, health care in America, compared with other wealthy and sophisticated countries, is abnormally expensive—a complete outlier. Second, for all that excess cost, our care isn't consistently better, and in many important respects it's average or worse. Third, the trends in the quality of our care are bad. On many of the measures of what we ultimately want from medical care—we've looked at safe children and long healthy lives—with each year we compare more and more unfavorably with our peers. What we see isn't other countries catching up to us as they grow in wealth, but other countries catching up, passing us, and leaving us behind.

Fathoming just how much *extra* we spend

Statistics having to do with the costs of medical care are like trillion dollar deficits: difficult to fathom. I won't try to build for you any piles of twenty-dollar bills that stretch to the moon and back, as I find those examples just as incomprehensible as the numbers themselves. Let's instead consider what else we might have purchased with the extra money we're spending on health care.

I find these comparisons helpful, as when we're not paying for health care directly with money that could be used for other things, its cost is just an abstract number. During my first term as governor, when we had to rein in Tennessee's Medicaid program I was trying to find a way to explain to the public (and first, to my Aunt Naomi) just how out-of-kilter things had become. The approach I took was to forget about anecdotes and comparisons with other states, and just describe how our TennCare costs compared with some of the other obligations of our state government.

Here's a couple of examples that I used. In TennCare, in 2004, the cost of the pharmacy benefit alone—the prescriptions that the doctors wrote and our Medicaid members filled at the drug store—was greater than what the taxpayers spent on Tennessee's entire higher education system. The spending on the single drug that topped our pharmacy spending list—the antipsychotic drug Zyprexa—was greater than our entire contribution to the University of Tennessee Medical School. I believe comparisons like those brought home to Tennesseans just how expensive this health care program had become. A lot of reasonable people who were sympathetic to funding health care looked at those numbers, shook their heads, and said, "That doesn't make sense."

Incidentally, the Zyprexa comparison illustrates how many places there are in our health care system where we can contain costs. Zyprexa is a drug made and heavily promoted by Eli Lilly and Company. It's FDA approved for schizophrenics and patients with bipolar disorder. It's a powerful drug and some psychiatrists I consulted told me that it was a useful part of their arsenal in dealing with difficult cases. But in 2004, the approval for treating bipolar disorder had just recently occurred, and it was hard for me to believe that we had remotely as many patients in TennCare with schizophrenia as the numbers of prescriptions would imply. Our analysts looked more deeply into what was happening, and found that large numbers of Zyprexa prescriptions were being written, often by family practitioners, for conditions far from those for which it was FDA approved. It was being prescribed for dementia and sometimes being used as a sleeping pill. This gross overuse of the drug was a cost issue, of course, but it was a real quality of care issue as well.

In this same style, let's do a thought experiment on the national level with our Medicare and Medicaid programs. We'll look at them over the next twenty years. There are good federal projections for the cost of these programs for the next ten years, and the following ten we can just trend at the historical long-term rates of growth. We'll do this with the pre–Affordable Care Act numbers, as they're easier to project and will be more conservative anyway.

Let's imagine we're going to make a serious effort to start bringing these costs under control and our goal will be to stop them growing as a percentage of our GDP. If we're at 17% today, we're going to find ways to keep our expenditures pinned there for the next twenty years. The number of dollars we spend each year will continue to grow, but at the rate of our economy and not faster. At the end of the twenty years, we'll still likely be more expensive than our peers (if we had done this for the last twenty years, we'd today still be the highest in the OECD). This thought experiment plan is not an overly aggressive one.

We'll take the official projections for the next ten years and combine those with some reasonable projections about what happens in the second ten. When we do that, we'll find that our strategy will produce total savings over what we would have spent of about $20 trillion over the twenty years, and that the present value of those savings will be about $9 trillion. Now this is an astonishing amount of money, so just to get an idea of how much, let's spend some of it.

I've never liked coal-fired electrical generation very much. There's all that carbon contributing to global warming. To get the coal, we shave off the tops of mountains, tear up the landscape, and permit miners to die in mine accidents. We build huge piles of ash we'll have to do something with someday. Here's a fantasy: let's, over the next twenty years, replace every single coal burning electric generation plant in America with nuclear power. (Don't worry, this is just a thought experiment; we won't actually build these in your backyard). To do so would take about 250 new nuclear plants (and, of course, create a huge number of jobs in the process). Could we at least make a down payment on this strategy with some of those savings from lowering the growth rate in Medicare and Medicaid? Actually, we could make a lot more than a down payment; all of that new nuclear power plant construction would use about 8% of the savings. 92% to go.

While I don't care for coal, I *am* a big fan of renewable energy generation, especially solar energy. To provide for growth, let's add fifty gigawatts of round-the-clock equivalent capacity here, about the equivalent of forty-two additional nuclear plants. To do this with wind and solar, we have to build about five times that average capacity because of clouds and night and calm days, or about another 250 gigawatts of capacity. This is especially valuable power, as a lot of it comes online when demand is high, and so it can substitute for expensive peak-demand capacity. With some conservative assumptions about the cost of these things in the future, we can do this with about another 8% of the savings. We're up to 16% now, and we've brought the cost of power to our consumers and factories down a lot because we've already paid the large capital costs of these technologies. With solar in particular, once you've built the arrays, the power is almost free for the transportation.

We still have lots of money to spend from these savings. Let's pick another capital project, one that, whatever your view of its merits, seems in any case very expensive: high-speed rail. We'll build ten thousand miles of new high-speed rail lines, and connect most of the larger urban areas of the nation. At the average $50 million per mile that the proposed California high-speed rail project costs, that will absorb another 6%. We've still used less than a quarter of the savings from our admittedly modest strategy, so we can keep going. If we think we're going to be upset when the

Chinese are looking outward from their moon base while we're spending our money on more Zyprexa, we need to use perhaps another 5% of the savings to get there first. And so on.

The federal deficit

The point of our thought experiment is simply to put in perspective the huge amount of clearly excess cost that we've allowed to infect our health care system. When we tackle this problem—and it's absolutely "when" and not "if," as we have no choice—in reality we couldn't divert the savings to build clean energy power plants or high-speed rail. We'll need it all just to help bring our country's finances under control. It's fair to say that our deficit problem can't be solved without solving the Medicare and Medicaid cost issues. The growth of these two programs alone and the federal underwriting of their solvency continues to make a deficit solution more difficult and painful each year.

Controlling our health care costs is an important national goal. Health care costs in the private sector are increasingly painful and compromise our competitiveness, but ultimately are self-limiting. Companies have to make profits, nonprofits have to balance their budgets, and they'll all do what it takes to accomplish what they need to or go out of business. But in the public sector, the reckoning is more distant. The borrowing that supports our lifestyle—including our health care expenses—doesn't magically create wealth any more than pumping oil out of a well creates more oil. We're such a rich country that the borrowing can go on for quite a while. But that borrowing, despite all the economists' mumbo jumbo, is nothing more than a mortgage on the future productivity of our nation. We're wealthy as a people, and this generation's borrowing taps a deep well, but it does have a bottom.

It's as if a fine family business has been created by the hard work of generations. Then, in this generation, along comes a young man who wants a fancy lifestyle but doesn't want to pay for it with his work. So he decides to simply borrow: to mortgage the assets of the business and take loans against its future earnings. He can do that for a while, and he can even appear very prosperous as he does so. But in the end he hollows out that proud family business and leaves it, deeply compromised, to his own sons and daughters. We're doing no different with the country we've inherited today.

Even the way we talk about deficits has changed. For the first part of my adult life, our nation ran some deficits, but they were modest. When we talked about government spending, a balanced budget was at least the norm. Balancing budgets was what we "should" do and the deficit spending had to be justified by the special needs of the day. Now it's quietly become very different. The norm is a budget with a large deficit, and those who place a high priority on returning to balance are "deficit hawks," political outliers who have to explain their concerns. The president's bipartisan commission has a goal of proposing ways to reduce the deficit to only the amount of the interest payments on our debt: roughly a half trillion dollars annually, and growing.

Here's one way I come to terms with just how much we're borrowing as a nation. In Tennessee, our general fund budget for the fiscal year 2010 is about $10 billion. We collect that amount in taxes from our citizens and businesses. It's a lot of money, and those taxes are a significant fact of life for both consumers and businesses in our state.

With the tax money we collect, we conduct our state's business. We operate a public school system with more than seventeen hundred schools and a higher education system of universities, community colleges, and technology centers. We operate a state prison and parole system. We pay our multibillion dollar share of the costs of Medicaid and a number of other federal programs. We operate a broad range of additional services for citizens with mental health needs and developmental disabilities. We pay for the mechanics of state government—our court system, legislature, district attorneys and public defenders, and dozens of regulatory agencies. We operate a law enforcement system with our highway patrol and the Tennessee Bureau of Investigation and we maintain an award-winning state park system. The past couple of years have been tough, and we've had to make painful cuts and watch the pennies. Our budget is constitutionally required to be balanced. We can't borrow for any operating purposes and any shortfalls have to be made up out of actual savings that we've put away in better times.

In 2010, while we're doing all these things, our federal government will borrow about $1.7 trillion to pay for things Congress has spent money on without arranging for the revenue to cover them. Some of this borrowing will come from the Social Security Trust Fund, and every dollar of those borrowings is a lien on the future earnings of every American. Tennessee is about 2% of the United States, and so our share of these borrowings is about 2% of that $1.7 trillion, or about $34 billion.

Think about this. Here in Tennessee, our share of the federal government borrowing, how much our own citizens have signed for, is *more than three times* our total state general-fund budget. Remember, this isn't the whole federal budget, just how much it's out of balance. Our national financial situation has become absurd. We've had a string of Congresses and administrations, of both parties, acting like an improvident couple who will buy and sign for anything they want, so long as they think they can keep up the monthly payments for a while. Anyone with a calculator can figure out that we can't grow out of this, and that there's no solution that doesn't go through major alterations to our spending on health care entitlements. That's why the Affordable Care Act, which deals with this problem by looking the other way, is such a disappointment.

Why health care costs so much

Now it's time to get to the heart of the problem: why does health care cost so much? Why is it so immune to the forces that create value and efficiency in other parts of our economy? Is there a new angle that will let us get a better look at the underlying problem? Let's do another thought experiment.

Let's take a trip together to our local supermarket, but with a difference. We'll pick up our cart and walk up and down the aisles putting things in our basket. Different employees of the supermarket—honest and well-meaning people, but on commission—will walk with us from time to time, making recommendations about things they think we need. Sometimes they'll just put something in our basket. There are lots of attractive displays, and we've seen some of the products advertised on television. We fill up our basket and head for the checkout. When we get there, the clerk rings things up, but we'll never see any prices, we'll never see the total, and the final bill is just sent off—somewhere—never to be seen again.

We all know intuitively that a box of oatmeal would cost twenty dollars in that supermarket, and that our shopping cart would have a lot more in it than it does in the real world. The reason is that in that hypothetical supermarket, the normal economic tension that helps us make choices and maximize value has been eliminated. When we visit an ordinary grocery store, we see the prices, we know that at the checkout we're going to have to pay, and we make choices that represent our values. We choose between steak and hamburger, we choose among brands and between brand-name and store-brand products, we don't put things in our basket that we don't want or plan to use. We even choose between spending money on items in the grocery store and other things we could do with the money like buying new clothes or taking a vacation.

There is a long litany of reasons offered for the high cost of health care—technology, drug companies, lifestyles, and on and on. But the simple fact is that health care has become very much like that grocery store. As more and more health care is paid for anonymously, through an obsolete insurance paradigm, the economic tension that creates value becomes weaker and weaker. A market economy needs tension, and we've systematically eliminated it.

When a doctor orders a test or a drug, performs a procedure or even just refers the patient elsewhere, she's doing so in a world where the normal economic give and take has been pushed deep into the background. The operation is performed, the drug dispensed, a referral made, and neither the patient nor the doctor has reason to care much about the cost. The bill is sent to some third party for payment, and there is only the most tenuous of connections between what is done to the patient and what the patient experiences through the insurance system. A million claims for services are bundled together and the insurance company actuary adjusts the rates accordingly. The patient and his employer, or the government, gets a little bigger bill for health insurance. There are no choices that he or even his doctor can make that will, by themselves, affect what comes out of his paycheck each month.

Of course, someone eventually has to pay, and that someone is still the patient: through a lesser wage than he might otherwise receive, through higher taxes, or through diminishing his children's economic prospects with federal borrowing. But those costs are very distant, and the connection with what is going on right now is hard to see. When the benefit is now and the costs are distant, we humans don't do very well—think of credit cards, or creative mortgages, or a loaded baked potato.

This is the nub of the problem, and putting our finger on it is the first step to figuring out how to create value—low cost and high quality—in our health care system. *The reason that health care costs so much is that we have systematically removed the tension between buyer and seller that makes economics work.*

- Patients don't care, because health insurance isolates them from the transaction and spreads costs so widely that they lose any connection to a particular transaction.

- Providers don't care, because when they're buyers they have no economic stake in the transaction. When they're sellers, they have an economic stake, but it's in the other direction.
- Insurance companies don't care. While they all have rules and checks to try to control costs, it's an administrative function and not really their money they're working with. They're financial intermediaries who pass on the actual costs, after they've done what they can, to another party.

We end up with a classic inelastic economic system. When the volume doesn't depend much on the price—which is the case in health care because the buyer doesn't feel the price—the optimum strategy for the seller is to keep increasing it. If you can increase the volume—the utilization of health care services—while you're at it, even better.

Creating tension by involving the patient

One approach that has been tried over the years to bring economic tension into play has been to engage the patient directly by making her responsible for a portion of the costs. For a long time now, health insurance plans have used co-pays ($25 for a doctor visit or a prescription, for example) and coinsurance (the patient pays 20% of the bill) as a way of engaging the patient economically. The most recent incarnation of this strategy has been the interest in Health Savings Accounts (HSAs). In this model, a consumer has a high-deductible health insurance policy to protect him from very expensive illnesses and a separate account that's typically funded with the difference between the lower cost of a high-deductible plan and the cost of a traditional health insurance plan. The patient then pays for the routine costs of health care out of this HSA account, and so in theory has a direct economic incentive to manage these costs carefully, both to prevent exhausting the account and, ideally, to build up savings for future medical expenses. The HSA was given a significant boost in the Medicare Modernization Act of 2003 by allowing contributions to these accounts to be made without taxes being paid on them.

A fundamental shortcoming of these cost-sharing approaches is that they all rely to some degree on the ability of a patient to make careful and informed purchasing decisions when it comes to medical care. This is very difficult: the practice of medicine by its nature requires great knowledge and expertise as well as a trusting relationship between the patient and the doctor. The patient doesn't have, and shouldn't be expected to have, the ability to make an informed judgment as to whether some medical service is needed in the first place.

Once a physician orders a service for his patient, the idea that the patient will then carefully compare price and quality to get the best deal may be theoretically interesting but is far from how it actually works. Even if a patient has the time, the technical skills, and the inclination to start down this road, any individual health care purchase is likely a part of a larger package that can't be predicted in advance. If my doctor refers me to a specialist for some nonemergency reason, it's just conceivable that I might research the fees and the quality reports and make a choice. I'd be far more likely, though, to simply take my doctor's advice. Even if I do the research, and choose a specialist, when she examines me and tells me the next step is an MRI and some lab tests, what do I do then? Will I next research each of those as well? Medical care is not cut and dried and one thing often leads to another; it is a far messier process than checking out the deals and reviews before buying a television or a cell phone.

More importantly, it's also a much more emotional process. Much of the truly expensive medical care occurs in the context of an emergency or a serious illness, and here the paradigm of the informed consumer making careful choices falls apart completely. If my son or wife were ever to be brought to the hospital with a serious medical problem, I know how I'd feel: scared and emotional. I feel certain that starting to rationally compare prices and quality for whatever treatment was appropriate would not be high on my list of things to do. If I were ever to find myself in the emergency room with severe chest pains and the doctor were to tell me that I need a stent, or open heart surgery, my first impulse would not be to hop on a computer and check prices. These are the times when we all need what doctors have always provided their patients—reassurance, help, and their expertise—not a comparison shopping assignment on the Internet.

Lastly, the patient's "skin in the game" has to come to an end somewhere, and that's a final serious weakness. Nearly every approach for financially involving the patient puts a cap on his obligation, typically a few thousand dollars or a percentage of his income. After that the insurer picks up the whole cost. That's a reasonable and necessary financial protection for individuals and families. Even if that protection wasn't there, there's the practical limitation that individual patients don't have unlimited resources. At some point their savings are gone and their credit limits exceeded (and the poor may have neither of these) but we're not going to stop their health care. Since a great deal of the real cost in medical care is in relatively few people with expensive episodes, just when we most need whatever influence consumer-driven care can offer, it's inevitably pinched off and we're back to plain old first-dollar coverage for everything.

There's a role for consumer participation in paying for health care, but we need to recognize that it's a limited tool and doesn't have an effect in the areas where the big costs occur. When the care that's being considered is truly elective, some financial participation by the patient can help manage costs. It's a way to create some economic tension and place that care in the context of other things that patient might like to do with the money. If a patient wants a Cesarean section, not for her health or the health of the baby, but for convenience, it's reasonable and effective to ask her to bear a share of the cost. If she has a heart attack, her financial participation in the resulting medical care is meaningless.

Creating tension by involving doctors

If involving patients more fully in paying for their health care doesn't work as well as we'd like in controlling costs, perhaps bringing providers themselves more into the equation is the solution. A variety of ways have been proposed to do this. The Affordable Care Act specifically authorizes a variety of pilot projects to explore the potential of alternative payment systems and experimenting with these has been an important part of discussions of health reform over the past quarter of a century.

Health maintenance organizations (HMOs) were designed around one such alternative payment system: the concept of "capitating" providers. What this term means is that a provider is given a fixed payment each month for each person (each "head") for whom they agree to provide any medical services needed by that patient in their area of expertise. A primary care provider would be given a monthly payment for each patient for whom they agree to provide primary care. A group of obstetricians would receive a payment for each woman who is enrolled with them. This arrangement has two purposes. First, it eliminates all the insurance billing arrangements of a fee-based system and the substantial administrative costs that entail. There are no price lists, claims, or reimbursement checks, just one monthly check to a provider to do what is necessary for each of the enrolled patients. Second, and more central to the concept, the provider's incentives change. She no longer has any financial incentive to perform more services as she's paid the same whether or not those services are performed.

I was an executive of an HMO in the 1980s and worked hard to find ways to make capitation work; it is devilishly difficult. The first problem was that almost any arrangement we could contrive had unintended consequences. With physician care, for example, we tried in some areas to capitate the primary care physicians and then pay negotiated fee-for-service rates to the various specialty providers. It seemed like a good idea, placing the primary care physician in the dual roles of both a provider of basic care for a fixed, agreed-upon price and an independent expert consultant on when and where referrals needed to be made. The unintended consequence, which I should have foreseen, was that the incentives favored primary care physicians spending little time with their patients—they were already being paid all that they were going to get—and instead referring every problem they could to specialists. Even with negotiated specialist rates, costs went up not down.

To address these issues, we also tried arrangements where the primary care physician received a capitation, but also had an economic stake in the cost of the referrals. That typically took the form of establishing a pool of money to pay for referrals, and then giving the physicians a share of any excess money or billing them a share of any shortfall at the end of the year. This created the problem of encouraging the behavior for which HMOs are frequently criticized: the underutilization of medical care. The primary care physicians did cut down on unneeded referrals. Unfortunately they also cut down on needed referrals.

The third obvious alternative—capitation agreements for everyone—didn't solve the problem either. It was frequently impossible in all but the largest urban areas. If there's one group of obstetricians in a community, they probably have little interest in a capitation arrangement. What we all learned in the HMO field was that capitation agreements by themselves often didn't do very much. If the underlying behavior of the physicians didn't change, the capitation agreements just ended up paying high costs more efficiently.

Capitation arrangements also often presented the HMOs with a business difficulty. When providers made money with them, they congratulated themselves and deposited their checks. However, most physician practices are professional corporations and pay nearly all their income directly to the physicians without establishing reserves and equity like a business might. If the group comes out behind, their share of the losses comes, very visibly and painfully, out of their personal checking accounts. What results is an angry physician group demanding an increase in their payments so that it doesn't happen next year. Sometimes a group threatens to quit unless you fix the problem right now. I don't describe this to elicit sympathy for the plight of the poor HMO corporation but it's evidence that in any incentive arrangement that works, there are winners and losers, and the response of the losers has to be taken into account.

While managed care hasn't proved to be the magic solution that many hoped it would be twenty-five years ago, there are lessons to be learned from the experience. It's had some successes, and well-run HMOs provide health care to highly satisfied customers in many parts of the United States. To do so, they have developed, over time, relationships with their providers that work for both sides. One of the lessons of the managed care experience, however, is that there are definite limits to what can be achieved simply with provider incentives. Furthermore, what works with one provider group in one community may be nothing like what works with another elsewhere. The culture and dynamics of the medical community in one place is likely to be very different from that in another. One size definitely doesn't fit all.

There are other approaches to financial arrangements with providers as well. One being widely discussed today is the concept of "bundled payments," which is a variation of sorts on what capitation tries to do. With this payment methodology, there's a fixed payment for a given episode of service that covers all of the various items necessary to perform it. If an orthopedic surgeon tells me that I need spinal surgery for back pain, my insurer might use a bundled payment concept to pay for it. That means that all the costs of my care—hospital payments, surgeon's and anesthesiologist's fees, various ancillary services such as laboratory and imaging, follow-up visits, perhaps some home health care—will be lumped into a single payment. That approach to payment has some advantages: it is simple to administer, and it gives the manager of the process, typically a hospital, the incentive to control the overall cost of the procedure. It reins in outliers: a surgeon whose fees are above the community norms is likely to be brought back to the center.

But it also misses a lot, starting with the basic question of whether the surgery is warranted at all. I used the example of bundling payments for back surgery as it's an expensive and notoriously overused procedure. Being able to control the price better and perhaps reducing it a few percent is good, but avoiding an unnecessary surgery altogether is far better. By itself, the technique of bundling payments does nothing to address this far larger issue.

Over the past quarter of a century we've tried to reengage economic forces by creating incentives in the existing payment systems. We have had, at best, modest success with this, but shouldn't be surprised. If the CEO of a large and complex organization tried to manage its operations primarily through setting up complex financial incentives for every employee of the company and then setting things on autopilot, we'd just laugh. We know that he'd never get the incentives right everywhere and there would be all sorts of unintended consequences. Managing cost and quality will take a much deeper toolbox. Most of all, it will take a change in the structure of the medical care system in a way that has every participant seeing a connection between their own interests and the goals of the organization.

The bottom line

Isolating and describing clearly why health care costs so much is the pivot around which the ideas in this book revolve. You, as the reader, may or may not agree with my critique of reform or my thoughts on fixing the problems that follow in the pages ahead. But boring in to find the core issue is the way to start solving complicated problems, and if you take nothing else from this book, I'd like you to remember this:

Our high cost of health care, and its continued high rate of growth, is not the result of technology, or administrative overhead, or chronic disease, or malpractice suits, or the lack of information systems, or transparency. It's the direct and inevitable result of our having systematically removed the economic tension between buyer and seller that makes efficient markets work. Health care has plenty of sellers who want what all sellers want: high volume and high prices. What's lacking is buyers who have a reason to care.

Patients are insulated from that tension by the mechanics of insurance; remember our grocery store. Providers have no incentives to manage external costs and every incentive to increase their own. Insurance companies are first of all financial intermediaries who accurately pass costs on. Managing them is secondary.

We've reached our second stepping-stone and identified the problem we have to solve: how do we ethically and intelligently reintroduce economic tension into health care? How do we put our economic system back to work for us? If it's difficult to restore economic tension through individual patients or health care providers themselves, the obvious question is: where and how *can* this tension be created? Solving this problem is the subject of the next few chapters.

8

Stepping-Stone Three: Managing Hypercomplexity

. . . in which we describe a new management challenge
in hypercomplex systems such as American health care.
We look at two other hypercomplex systems: market
economics and natural selection. We look for the
underlying mechanisms that make them work
and identify a three-step cycle that is at the heart of
the matter. We consider how to apply that cycle to
our health care system, and conclude that the key lies
in a robust and comprehensive approach to defining
and measuring quality.

Many years ago, when I was in college, I read a book by Richard
Neustadt, *Presidential Power*. At one point in it, he describes Truman talking about the frustrations that he expects Eisenhower to
face as president. "He'll sit here," Truman would remark, "and
he'll say 'Do this! Do that!' *And nothing will happen. Poor Ike. It
won't be a bit like the army. He'll find it very frustrating.*"

His point was that in deep and highly complex organizations—
the United States government in this case—by the time orders get
down into the places where the actual execution takes place, they're

a long distance from where they were given in the first place. The connection is weak and the consequences of failing to follow an order often modest. What started out as an order is diluted to become just one of many incentives and pressures that bear on the person who has to carry it out. The sum of all these various incentives can easily be unrelated or even contrary to the original purpose for which the order was given.

In some cases, of course, orders from the top work. When President Obama fired General McChrystal, as President Truman did General MacArthur, that general is fired. Neustadt says that this kind of order has the four characteristics that ensure its execution: the president has the clear authority to give it, the order itself is unambiguous, it is easy to tell if the order has been carried out, and the consequences of failing to do so are severe.

But the vast majority of even a president's orders are not like that at all. Our government is one of shared powers, and the essence of the power of its chief executive is the power to persuade, not to order.

At the other extreme from firing a general, suppose the president wants to fulfill a campaign promise and make the employees who work in Human Services offices around the country treat their clients with more helpfulness and respect. He makes his wishes very clear and orders his HHS secretary to make it happen. At the Human Services office in a county somewhere in the Midwest, a woman who interviews these clients may be very aware that the president wants something, although she likely has already received multiple mixed messages as to exactly what that is. The evening news had a report on the president's actions that irritated her considerably, she has a boilerplate e-mail that went to a large distribution list from her state director, and the supervisor in her office has been talking with them about why the president doesn't really understand what they actually do.

Whatever her interpretation of the president's stated intentions, in the end they're not a large part of the incentives that bear on her day-to-day conduct. She had a fight with her husband last night, there's a particularly difficult and abusive client waiting to see her, she has civil service protection and is unlikely to be fired for any reason other than gross misconduct, there are regulations as to what she can and cannot say to a client that aren't necessarily consistent with what the president wants, she isn't seeking promotion, and her own concept of professionalism is more oriented to efficient and accurate determination of eligibility than to customer service. The president and his desires, or orders for that matter, are a long way away and her behavior is much more influenced by things that are very local and immediate.

In Neustadt's terms, the president's actions fail all the tests for a self-executing order: the president's authority isn't completely clear. The order is ambiguous. Neither the president nor anyone remotely near him will ever know if she carried out what he wanted. The consequences of failing to do so are not severe, and in fact the consequences to things she cares about may be worse if she does.

The insight that I took from Neustadt's book was that there is really no such thing as an order or a rule. *Everything* is persuasion. Every individual is at every point constantly evaluating a variety of pressures and incentives that bear on any action they might take. All you can ever do is to alter some of that surrounding environment and try to shift the sum of all those incentives closer to what you want them to do.

Sometimes the incentive you create is very strong: when President Truman fired General MacArthur, the cost of refusing the president's action would likely have been public and professional disgrace or even a prosecution for treason. But the order is not absolute, he *could* have refused: his reputation and standing with the military establishment and the public was such that a refusal might just conceivably have held. Perhaps the president would have had to back down, or Congress might have chosen to impeach the president over the situation. I presume that these ideas at least crossed the mind of the proud general of the army, but that in the summing-up, the consequences of refusal to his reputation and innate patriotism far outweighed the benefits.

Of course, most of the incentives and pressures we create in organizations are much more modest. If someone who works for me refuses a direct order, I can fire them, but that's hardly the worst thing that could ever happen and certainly insufficient to get them to do something criminal or reprehensible to their values. I can set up financial incentives, and they can have an effect, but financial incentives frequently fail to overcome peer pressure or professional pride, not to mention laziness or hostility.

The underlying thought here is straightforward: that the laws and rules and policies we use to manage behavior are not in any sense absolute, they are only persuasive. Whatever effect they have is in the context of all the other pressures and incentives in a person's environment. As organizations get larger and more complex, the distance from the organization's policy makers gets greater and greater, the ability to impose structure from the top gets weaker and weaker, and the local environment becomes a larger and larger factor in the summing-up of every pressure that results in someone's behavior.

Organizations

This chapter is about organizations. We periodically go through disillusionment about the way in which organizations function and we're in one such period right now. But the reality is that they're the vehicle that society uses to accomplish tasks. We all have a sense of what they look like, in part because many of us spend our days working in one. Modern corporations, for the most part, produce and deliver goods and services efficiently and non-profit organizations provide needed cultural and social services in a community. A modern governmental organization can conduct wars or build roads. A great deal of attention has been given to the management of these organizations. Magazines and journals abound and there are entire sections in bookstores devoted to topics such as marketing, finance, strategy, operations research, and the development of human capital. Many of the best and brightest of our young people have devoted their careers to the science of designing and managing organizations to carry out tasks that are important to society.

In most parts of our economy, the structure stops there. America has a vast array of restaurants, newspapers, retail stores, hotels, colleges and universities, construction companies, orchestras, museums, and on and on. Each of these areas incorporates a great diversity of organizations: large and small, public and private, for-profit and nonprofit, union and nonunion, well-run and poorly run. The individual pieces have great variety in how they see their mission: among universities there's Harvard and Bob Jones, there's the San Francisco Art Institute and the Massachusetts Institute of Technology. That very diversity is one of the reasons for the success of our economy. As a nation, we're not trying to organize them to any larger purpose—there's no call for a national restaurant policy, and, to the best of my knowledge, Congress is not considering museum reform—because we're not paying for these things centrally and we don't see a compelling national interest in a common purpose. The individual pieces remain relatively small, at least compared to the national economy, and traditional management and organizational science works well for them.

Health care isn't like that. It's not just large, it's vast. We pay for a great many of the services it provides centrally and have a direct and legitimate interest in the cost and quality of those services. There's a genuine national interest in ensuring that our citizens have good health care.

Hypercomplex organizations

We all relate to the problem that Richard Neustadt was describing. Who hasn't been discouraged or angered by the inertia and inability to get things done in big and complex organizations? Our frustration is often directed at government, which by its very nature is both big and complex. Depending on your ideological disposition, you might blame indifferent bureaucrats, unions, incompetent politicians, greedy corporations, or a long list of other reasons.

I want to offer a different culprit: that when systems grow past a certain point of size and complexity, the way they work inherently changes, new kinds of behavior emerge, and we need a different approach to the problem of getting them to do what we want. I'm going to call these "hypercomplex" systems and the American health care system is a good example. As our society grows more complex, these hypercomplex systems will play an increasingly important role in the way we get the big things done—like better organizing health care. Instead of beating our fists against the wall of their unresponsiveness to the traditional ways we manage things, we need to just recognize that they're different. They don't work like the organizations we're used to, and if we plan to use them to accomplish our ends, we need a new branch of management science.

The defining characteristic of a hypercomplex "organization" is that on a large scale it's not organized, it's amorphous: it's more of a *collection* of varied pieces than a coherent structure assembled out of those pieces. The individual pieces are diverse, only loosely tied together, and largely march to their own drummer. That is a good description of our health care system.

American health care has little structure: it's a collection of a large and diverse set of players. Our roughly eight hundred thousand physicians do their work in a huge variety of physician practices: big, small, and solo; single specialty and multispecialty; salaried and fee-for-service. There are thousands of hospitals, ranging from rural community hospitals with ten or twenty beds to complex urban teaching institutions with many hundreds of beds and thousands of employees. They're organized as for-profits and nonprofits and there are general hospitals and those devoted to specific specialty areas. There are outpatient clinics, dialysis centers, surgery centers, and home health agencies. These providers of care are supported by an array of companies providing products such as drugs and medical equipment and services such as laboratory testing and information technology. Medical care is paid for by individuals, by employers, and by government at every level.

The individual goals of the various pieces are often quite different and aren't necessarily aligned to any overarching goals we might try to designate. Every piece of the health care system that I've described shares at some level the goal of providing medical care, but there are many views of what that means and many other and, often more imperative, goals as well. Doctors and nurses are human, they want to make money and they gravitate to places and areas of medicine that make that possible. Hospitals are interested in organizational success and self-preservation. Companies have shareholders and exist as businesses to deliver profits.

The problem at hand is to try and figure out how to make our health care system more responsive to our goal of delivering high quality health care as efficiently as possible. This has proved difficult so far. Perhaps a starting place is to step back and view what we have from a different angle; to see our health care system—our hypercomplex system—as fundamentally different from the smaller organizations of our experience and responsive to a different set of rules. When we do so, the next question is how we might find out what those rules are.

Two other hypercomplex systems

Not surprisingly, there are examples of what I term hypercomplex systems all around us; it's the way most of the world works. Our invention of organizations was a tool for us to simplify and put some structure around the complexity of human behavior and allow us to accomplish things that require the coordinated efforts of a lot of people. The underlying reality looks, however, much more like the hypercomplexity that I've described.

I'm going to take two hypercomplex systems that are right in front of us and see what we can learn from them: modern free-market economics and the operation of natural selection in the process of evolution. These are both extraordinarily complex systems that nevertheless work well (with, of course, plenty of exceptions). Our free-market economy produces a huge range of goods and services—steaks and airplane travel and iPods—and it does so efficiently and adaptly. The operation of natural selection—of evolution—produces a vast range of successful forms of life: bacteria and jellyfish and frogs and tigers and people who read books.

Both are worth studying carefully to learn how to better manage something as complex as our health care system. When we want, for example, to reduce the number of unnecessary services that a patient receives, we can try to set rules from the top. Medicare does this all the time. But if the powerful local incentives that a doctor feels—the economic advantage of providing more services, pressure from suppliers and other professionals, pressure from the patient, the doctor's own habits, the fear of lawsuits—drive his behavior in the opposite direction then it's no contest. The closer and more immediate incentives will win out every time.

The reason to look at free markets and natural selection is that they've solved this problem. They're adaptable, they optimize things, *and they do so almost entirely through the workings of local incentives rather than top-down structure.* (If you're either a communist or a creationist, you might want to skip to the next chapter.)

Market economics

Market economies are in some sense a human invention, but have deep roots in the way our minds work. We're social beings, and we've been wired to engage in economic transactions since before we were human. We've been interacting with our fellow humans and trading food, shelter, sex, tools, protection, and a great many other things for food, shelter, sex, tools, protection, and a great many other things for a very long time. Today, a good deal of this trading uses an invented tool for exchange—money. But when we go to work for a paycheck and then use the money to pay our rent and grocery bill with it, we're engaging in a modern version of transaction that has been going on for a long time.

One of the great strengths of any market economy is its adaptability. The world is a dynamic place and there are constant shifts in the landscape. Advances in technology, for example, make new things possible. When the technology of integrated circuits advances, we promptly get the Internet, personal computers, and iPods. When buggy whips are no longer necessary, the companies that make them disappear or move on to something else. There's no overarching plan here, nor is there anyone smart or prescient enough to write one if they wanted to. Rather, entrepreneurs and innovators find new niches and exploit changes, and things that are no longer wanted make way for those that are. Businesses prosper, hang on, or die based on the attractiveness, right now, of what they have to offer.

I recognize that there are many ways in which we wish that our market-based economic system worked differently. It doesn't always optimize just what we think it should. Right now, we're working through the throes of a deep recession caused in substantial part by the workings of a market-based financial system. It's hard, however, to blame today's woes on the mechanics of the market system itself. It responded very well—too well for our own good—to the presence of buyers who were mistakenly willing to pay for something without looking too closely. Sometimes they purchased bonds and sometimes houses, but our underlying economic system provided them with what they were willing to buy efficiently and quickly.

As a point of interest, there's a parallel in this failure of our financial system with the problem in health care we discussed in the previous chapter—the elimination of the economic tension between buyer and seller. The world became flooded with bad mortgages because Wall Street invented a way—the successful packaging of mortgage-backed securities for resale—to eliminate the economic tension that's always balanced the behavior of banks. When banks kept the mortgages they wrote, or sold them to known and careful buyers, they had two incentives working to keep everything in check. The banks wanted to write mortgages to earn fees and interest, but they also needed to be careful in assessing the ability for those mortgages to be repaid. Once half of that tension was removed—they could sell all the mortgages they wanted into a vast anonymous pool—the result was the unconstrained influence of the first incentive, and they wrote both good and bad mortgages at a great rate. Our health care system, under the skin, has some features very much like the financial system that has just so badly bitten us.

Natural selection

The second system that I want us to look at is the process of natural selection, the mechanics underlying the operation of evolution. While this might seem like an odd place to look for guidance in something as specific as health care, natural selection is adaptable and self-adjusting in just the way we are seeking. As with a market-based economy, it achieves its results not through overarching rules but in the way in which many small and individual events work.

This is probably not as familiar a subject as a market economy, so let's take a moment and review how it works. The characteristics of every living thing are determined by its genes; every gene is one small section of the DNA that we all know about. Genes are passed on from each generation to the next; that's what makes the offspring of an oak tree or a trout look like an oak tree or a trout.

Where it gets interesting is that every once in a while, one of the genes that's being passed on to the next generation undergoes a change that is called a *mutation*. That mutation might be caused by natural radiation or some chemical agent, and usually doesn't affect the organism itself (an exception would be a mutation that causes a cell to become cancerous). Since genes determine the characteristics of living things, the individual in that next generation with that altered gene is different in some way. Most of the time, the mutation hurts—there's a lot more ways for things to get worse than better. It diminishes the ability of the organism that carries it to live, compete, and produce offspring of its own. Descendants of that first mutated organism are on the whole a little less successful in producing the next generation than their competitors without the mutation, and the mutated gene declines and, likely, eventually extinguishes itself.

Once in a while, though, the trait created by the mutation allows its possessor in some way to prosper so that its chances of making descendants of its own are increased. If that happens, over many generations more and more individuals have that gene and the characteristic that it engenders. It comes into being as an accident, and over time becomes more and more prevalent than the unmutated one. The species has some new characteristic that has become well established and a tiny piece of evolution has occurred. To take a specific example, let's think about a finch, a bird that eats seeds for a living and was studied by Charles Darwin. Perhaps a mutation occurs, and a finch is born with a beak a little longer than that of the other finches. This will likely make some difference in its ability to survive, find a mate, and have offspring of its own. Perhaps the new, longer beak hurts by making it just a little bit harder to get away from a predator. In that case, the particular "experiment" in longer beaks just didn't work out and that mutated gene declines and disappears. But perhaps, while the bigger beak still makes it a little bit harder to escape a predator, it's more efficient enough in getting at the seeds it eats that it grows larger and healthier. It can compete for a mate better. In that case, the net effect of the longer beak is that the lucky finch is more successful in producing offspring. The gene will grow in the population and eventually the whole population of finches will have longer beaks.

More than anything else, the operation of natural selection makes life adaptable. Perhaps our finches live on an island and they've reached the sweet spot for beak length—not too short and not too long—and now a few of them are blown by a storm to a different island, one normally isolated from their original home. On this new island, the plants that are the source of the finches' seed food are a little different, and the seeds are deeper in their cones than the ones back home. The equilibrium changes, bigger beaks have a greater advantage, and the length of finch beaks grows to reach a new balance at a larger size.

The common features of hypercomplexity

The parallels between a market economy and natural selection should be clear at this point, and there are four points about these two hypercomplex systems that I want to emphasize.

First, to operate well, they need an environment where resources are limited, where's there's not room for everything. If everyone's as rich as they want to be, there's little incentive to innovate and produce new goods and services. If the finches live in a finch Garden of Eden of limitless resources and no predators, it doesn't matter much just what size their beak is.

Second, both hypercomplex systems are very good at continuously optimizing something. In the case of a market economy, it finds an optimum price that best balances the interests of the buyer and seller. If it were higher, the seller would like it better but the buyer would be less inclined to buy; if it were lower, the buyer would be happier, but the seller less inclined to part with what he has to sell. In the case of natural selection, nature finds an optimum beak length for our finch that maximizes its ability to survive and create new finches. It finds an equilibrium length that best balances its ability to escape predators with the need to find food.

Third, they're self-adjusting when changes occur. The equilibrium that these hypercomplex systems achieve in price or beak length is transitory because the real world is always in motion. In a market economy, the price of materials, the weather, technology, and the preferences of consumers change constantly and often quickly. In nature, new predators with new capabilities show up, weather patterns shift, and new species try to invade the ecological niche of food and shelter that our finches inhabit.

When these changes in the surroundings occur, the balance that has been achieved is upset, the incentives change slightly, and a new optimum is quickly found. We used to buy televisions with big and heavy picture tubes. Then something changed: new technology made flat panel televisions possible, consumers preferred them, and the business of manufacturing televisions shifted to the production of the new thing consumers wanted. Furthermore, it's not a one-dimensional adjustment. The mix and prices of plain old picture tube televisions and fancy new flat panels will change, but a great many other things will adjust as well. The new flat panels are attractive and consumers are willing to spend more of their entertainment dollars to buy one. The production and sales of stereo equipment adjusts downward slightly and television viewership goes up a little bit, and with the latter advertising rates go up as well. There are a million small adjustments, but no committees needed to meet, no laws were passed or rules made; the market for televisions just finds its new equilibrium.

Fourth, they operate through adding up small effects from many local incentives and not some overarching structure or plan. When the flat panel televisions hit the shelves, everyone doesn't immediately run out and buy one. Rather, the new flat panel televisions become just a little more desirable to the consumer and, as a result, slightly more often some consumer makes the decision to buy one instead of something else. That's just one tiny contribution to the growth of the flat panel market at the expense of other things, but when you sum the effect of millions of those little choices, the flat panel industry prospers and the old picture tube television industry declines. Our finch with the longer beak has just a little advantage in getting to food. Most of the time it doesn't make any difference, but when food is scarce or the competition for it is intense, the advantage of being a little better fed lets a male win the competition for a mate or a female be able to lay an extra egg. These little advantages, summed over time and lots of finches, result in more long-beaked finches and fewer regular-beaked ones.

Because the way market economies and natural selection work, through summing-up the effects of many smaller scale events, they have a huge advantage over traditional organizations—they scale. As they get bigger and more complex, they don't break down because the communication lines that determine their behavior get longer and noisier. The communication lines always stay short and local. It's just the opposite: they work better as they get larger and their behavior becomes more predictable.

The secret of managing hypercomplexity

This book is about health care, not organizations. We're trying to figure out how to make a sprawling health care system respond to our wishes: so, what can we learn from hypercomplexity?

Here's the secret: the world has limited resources and there's lots of competition. Under the hood, our hypercomplex systems use a simple, three-step cycle, endlessly repeated, to compete for resources and adapt to change.

Step 1. There is a fluid source of variation in the environment.

Step 2. There is a simple metric, a simple measurement, that determines which of the many variations are better and which are worse.

Step 3. There is a way to help the better variations propagate and grow and weed out the worse ones.

Let's consider these simple steps one at a time.

A fluid source of variation. In a market economy, there are rich sources of new candidate products and services: entrepreneurs have ideas, inventors invent, scientists and engineers discover and develop new technologies. The preferences and needs of consumers are constantly in flux as values change and alternatives come into being. In the world of natural selection, there's a constant stream of mutations that alter characteristics. In both cases, this constant shaking up and experimentation at the lowest level is a lubricant; it allows many things to be tried and provides an unending stream of candidates to be tested against the status quo.

A metric. In a market economy, we use price to measure the value to us of some possible purchase. I'm a buyer faced constantly with a bewildering array of possible purchases, each with various advantages and disadvantages relative to the others. A very simple example: a cup of coffee is a product that comes in many variations. Starbucks competes with the gas station qwik-mart and coffee in fancy restaurants. I'm willing to pay a couple of dollars for a cup of coffee at Starbucks, but not at the gas station qwik-mart. The coffee beans are higher quality and the coffee tastes better, to me, at Starbucks. They have tables I can sit at and the place smells good but it's not so convenient and one of the baristas irritates me.

The qwik-mart variation I evaluate differently: the coffee is very convenient when I'm already buying gas and it's quick, but not as good. I'm not interested in paying two dollars for it, but a dollar is fine. Conversely, at the end of a meal in a fine restaurant, there's another variation: excellent coffee, a chance to extend a pleasant meal a little longer, china cups. That cup I sometimes value at four dollars. The advantages and disadvantages of each possibility are complex and hard to compare directly. My brain cuts through the complexity, summing up all the pluses and minuses, in its own way and deciding what something is worth to me with a simple measurement—the price I'm willing to pay.

With natural selection, the metric is equally one-dimensional: the number of little finches. If there is a variation to be evaluated— we've been talking about different beak lengths—all the possible advantages and disadvantages of one beak length versus another are summed up very simply: how many successful little finches does each one finally produce.

The secret of the success of these metrics, these measures of advantage or disadvantage, is that they're very simple. The effects that result from some variation—a new competitor in the coffee market or that longer finch beak—may be very complex, interrelated, and not obvious in their ultimate value. Market economies and nature don't give us a big spreadsheet, they distill it all down to a single number: the price I'll pay for a cup of Starbucks or the number of little finches in the next generation.

Propagate the good and weed out the bad. In a market economy, products and services that can command higher prices (relative to their cost to produce) are successful. They attract capital and talent, they spawn new variations and imitations, and their stockholders and the companies that make them prosper. Conversely, those products that don't measure up become starved for capital and talent, the companies that make them are not able to operate successfully, and decline. With natural selection and our finches, advantageous variations produce more offspring and disadvantageous ones fewer, and over time the genes that convey the advantage become more and more prevalent in the gene pool. That's why it's called natural *selection*.

This process of promoting or weeding out is not a right or wrong, yes or no proposition. There's always a mixture; variations that are really bad, sort of bad, neutral, sort of good, really good, and so on. Over time, however, this three-step cycle ensures that there is a steady drive toward finding the optimum in any environment: the optimum price for a cup of Starbucks and the optimum length of beak for a finch.

Application to our health care system

Looking at the American health care system in the light of this three-step process, we can start to see the problem. The first step—the presence of a source of variation, works well. Our American economy is inventive and flexible, and there is a constant flow of innovation in health care. We produce new drugs, new equipment, and new procedures on a regular basis. This part of the cycle works.

Let's skip for a moment to step three—mechanisms to grow the good and weed out the bad. Here things are more mixed. In some areas, there are powerful ways to eliminate things that don't work. When a pharmaceutical company introduces a drug that proves to be harmful, it's withdrawn, it diminishes the reputation of the company, and there is punishment in terms of lost profits, judgments against the company, and sometimes even fines. But much of health care is relatively immune from these selection pressures. There are an array of drugs and treatments that are clearly inferior to alternatives in the value or quality they deliver, and yet remain widely used. The institutions of medicine seem almost eternal: when did you last hear of a hospital going out of business for giving poor care or being inefficient?

Now let's come back to this second step—a metric, a way of valuing what we get. That's what's missing in health care.

Our health care system is hypercomplex and will continue to be highly resistant to management through top-down rules.

There's been no shortage of these in Medicare and Medicaid for almost fifty years and we've definitely discovered that they just don't work all that well. The answer is to drive health care decisions with that same three-step cycle that is at the core of other successful hypercomplex systems. The steering wheel of those systems is the metric. It specifies what's valued and what's not, and then innovation and feedback will drive the behavior of the system to that end. We need to invent a metric that's simple and incorporates our society's values about what our health care system should do for us.

The clear answer is that this metric ought to be *quality of care*. By that somewhat generic phrase I specifically mean the extent to which an episode of medical care is consistent with the best scientific information we have at the time and the best treatment. This is nothing more than the evidence-based medicine that's a staple of nearly every health care discussion.

Taking stock

This is our third stepping-stone—inventing a way to create the conditions that will induce our health care system to change in the ways we want. By looking at the way that other large, unorganized systems—other hypercomplex systems—work successfully, we can see the framework of an approach. We know we have to establish two things. First, we have to create an environment in which the total resources available are limited—that's what makes competition and selection work. In health care, that means closing down an open-ended system of reimbursement, setting an overall budget for what we're going to spend, and forcing the system to compete for those dollars. Second, we need to put the three-step cycle to work—innovations, a metric to value them, winners and losers. The key to engaging that cycle of innovation —the missing ingredient—is the metric, so we'll need to invent one and a robust way to define and measure it. The metric today in health care is vague. The way we're going to push health care in the direction we want is to tighten it up and make it about quality of care. Then we'll give it consequences—use it to produce some winners and losers.

Put most simply, we're going to make our health care system compete for a pool of money that has limits and we're going to dictate the terms of that competition to be about the needs of the patient and not the provider: to be about quality of care.

9

Stepping-Stone Four: Quality

... in which we define the quality metric that we need. We propose a way to create a comprehensive and accepted set of practice standards that reflect evidence-based medicine—our primary definition of quality. We discuss the right of patients to participate in decisions affecting them as a component of quality as well. We then create a "Red Book" to formally and explicitly define the standards and scoring we'll use in measuring quality.

To reach our fourth stepping-stone, I'm about to propose a considerable expansion of how quality of care is defined and assessed in our health care system. But before I start, I'd like to convince you that in doing so I'm not blundering around and messing up something that's working just fine, thank you.

Let me begin with a personal story. I recently toured the neonatal intensive care unit in a major hospital and met a young couple whose newborn baby had been brought there from a community hospital in a smaller city. Their little boy was struggling for his life. Her pregnancy had been without problems, and she had delivered the baby at her doctor's recommendation by scheduled Cesarean section about two and a half weeks before her due date. The baby was having severe problems breathing. This is a well-known possible complication with scheduled Cesarean section babies before thirty-nine weeks. It was her first baby (and the Cesarean section for this delivery meant that she would likely require one for any future child as well) and she and her husband were devastated. I checked back later, and the story ended well: the little boy survived, and went home after about three weeks in the NICU. At discharge, he had no observable impairments, but it can't be a good thing to spend your first days on Earth struggling to get enough oxygen.

The neonatal specialist physician told me the reason for the elective, early delivery. The mother's doctor had been about to leave for a vacation in the tropics and convinced her that this was the thing to do—unless, of course, she wanted to have the baby with whatever strange doctor happened to be on call. The couple trusted him and agreed to go ahead. Their little boy spent days with death or permanent damage a real possibility, the parents went through hell, the insurance company paid a quarter-million dollars or so, and the doctor presumably enjoyed his snorkeling.

There's no lawsuit here; the little boy went home with no obvious impairment. There's no likelihood of any professional discipline either; the delivery two and a half weeks early was within a window of time that until recently has been assumed to be safe.

But most Americans would see this as truly awful medical care.

This is a personal anecdote—a true one—but health care literature is full of well-documented examples of just how far medicine, as it's actually practiced, strays from evidence-based standards. In many cases, these disparities reflect a strong bias toward aggressive and lucrative intervention despite a lack of evidence that it can help, and often, in the face of evidence, are harmful.

Here's one recent sample. The Agency for Healthcare Research and Quality, which is an agency of the federal government within the Department of Health and Human Services, reported in 2009 on a study of 682 children on the use of surgically implanted ear tubes in children with middle ear infections. Compared to the existing published guidelines, 7.5% met the criteria and 93% did not. In case the existing guidelines were possibly outdated, they also had an expert panel write new ones for comparison; 7% of the surgeries were consistent with the updated standards.

This is in New York City, with a relatively sophisticated medical community. If 80% of the surgeries had met the guidelines, most reasonable people would easily assign the other 20% to that gray area where we defer to the professional judgment of the surgeon. When the surgeons are performing and getting paid for *fourteen times* the number of surgeries that professional standards call for, most reasonable people see a problem. This is partially a cost problem, but even more so a quality one. I believe we could all agree that a surgical procedure on a young child's middle ear is a really poor idea if it's not genuinely necessary.

The little boy in the NICU and the surgery on those New York children's ears are examples of poor quality caused by doing too much. There are also times when quality is hurt by doing too little —failing to perform services called for by evidence-based medicine. Many of these services are quite simple and inexpensive (which doubtless explains the relative lack of interest in performing them) but nonetheless have a large bearing on a patient's health.

The National Committee for Quality Assurance (NCQA) maintains scorecards on a number of quality indicators. These Healthcare Effectiveness Data and Information Set (commonly known as HEDIS) scorecards are full of examples of relatively simple but effective care procedures that are frequently omitted. Remember that the patients covered by these measures are by definition those *with* insurance—this is not about lack of care for the uninsured.

Some samples: children with sore throats should receive a strep-throat test before being prescribed antibiotics (this is not a cost saving measure because the antibiotics are relatively inexpensive; it's an important patient safety measure); the test is actually performed only about half the time. Eye exams are a standard and important part of the management of diabetes; nearly half of patients don't get them. Colon cancer is the second-leading cause of cancer-related death, and detection and treatment in its early stages is effective. There's virtually no debate that screening should be performed after age fifty: more than four out of ten don't get it. Quality assurance is a facet of our health care system that needs shaking up.

Evidence-based medicine

The concept of quality as it applies to medical care is intimately linked to the concept of "evidence-based" medicine and the extent to which the medical care actually being given corresponds to it. What most of us want from health care today is what people have always wanted: the benefit of the best medical science available to prevent illness, or when illness occurs, to cure it if possible, and to ameliorate its effects if it can't.

There's a lot of information to start with—a vast literature on the science and the effectiveness of various approaches to medical care. As in any field, some of it is excellent, some of it is useful, much of it is inconsistent, and doubtless some of it is junk. Medicine, however, is particularly prone to bias and sloppiness in research because so much of it is paid for or conducted by people with a strong economic interest in the results. In addition, the very volume of research is a significant problem in itself. It's become nearly impossible for any practitioner who is actually devoting most of her time to taking care of patients to keep up with all the research that bears on her daily decisions, let alone be asked to evaluate the quality of the research itself. There's a genuine disconnect in our health care system between the good information that's theoretically available and actually providing that information in a useable form to practitioners.

To reach our next stepping-stone, we need to set up a formal process to evaluate and distill the evidence we have about what constitutes the best medical care. We want a baseline national standard and we want that standard to be the highest in the world. Our understanding will always be changing and improving, so this needs to be a continuous process that relooks at everything frequently. Medicine is very complex, so we'll provide plenty of room for the intelligent judgment of the physician when it comes to deciding the best way to treat her patient.

Then we'll design a dashboard that defines what we'd expect to be able to measure from the outside if evidence-based care is being given. We'll design that dashboard in such a way that it can be used to calculate the simple quality metric that our strategy requires. Finally, we'll regularly publish all of this in an accessible format that can both guide the physician and be used to measure her against the profession's standards. This is not revolutionary. We're simply setting up in medicine the same kind of modern, effective quality-assurance system that works elsewhere in our economy.

When we build airplanes, we don't let every engineer and welder operate according to their own professional judgment and then check on the back end how often an engine fails or the plane crashes. Thankfully, we do it in real time. We set up standards and we make systematic checks against those standards throughout the whole process of designing and building the airplane. Quality measurement and checks should be embedded in the day-to-day operation of the health care system as well. When I go to my doctor with a problem, I'm not very interested in the national or regional statistics for how often that problem was treated correctly. I'm not even that interested in my own doctor's percentage score. I want to know that what is being done for *me,* this time, right now, is the best thing we know how to do.

American Medical Standards Panel

Establishing comprehensive practice standards is the starting point. This will be controversial, as physicians are understandably protective about their professional independence and prerogatives. It's hard to imagine, however, any real progress in improving quality without this starting point. If these standards can be set with complete professionalism and with the standing of support from both government and leaders in the professions themselves, it can be made to work.

The way to accomplish this it to set up what I'll call the American Medical Standards Panel (I'll call it the Standards Panel for short from here on). This Standards Panel should originate with the imprimatur of the federal government, separate and independent from the other health care activities of government. It'll be a stand-alone body, not buried in and inevitably compromised by the objectives or ideology of the Department of Health and Human Services or any other federal program. We want the considerations of this Standards Panel rooted in the profession of medical care and its membership should reflect that. It would consist primarily of men and women with professional health care expertise as physicians, scientists, or analysts. Representation by every interest group isn't necessary and isn't desirable. It will, of course, consider information and arguments brought to it by unions, insurance companies, professional groups, pharmaceutical companies, advocates, members of Congress, and a host of others. But its responsibility is the science—to establish, first of all, the standard of care from the point of view of the patient

This Standards Panel is not charged with evaluating the cost effectiveness of various alternatives. These judgments ultimately have to be made but we'll provide for them in another fashion later. They are welcome to comment on such differences where they consider it appropriate, but their core task is to put the interests of the patient first. The Standards Panel is the way in which the medical profession establishes the ideal standard for patient care—the goal toward which we strive within the operational and financial realities of the real world.

One of the keys to making this panel work is making sure that its funding is insulated from political pressure. The choices this panel will make will have large economic consequences for different interests and these interests are capable of bringing a great deal of pressure to bear. The Standards Panel would, of course, employ a staff to do much of the work, but this is not an expensive effort in the scheme of things. Its funding should not be an appropriation of any sort, but more independent. A modest fee on the various intermediaries in the health care system transmitted directly to them would be a workable solution. It would provide the needed insulation from interference that the panel will need to have any hope of success.

This independence of its budget from the political process is essential. Anyone who has served in an executive position in the public sector is well aware of how quickly and powerfully pressure is brought to bear through the budget process. There's an infamous example of such pressure in this very area of setting medical standards. Congress created the Agency for Health Care Policy and Research (AHCPR) in 1985 specifically to create evidence-based guidelines and to recommend to Medicaid and Medicare what items they should pay for. In the early 1990s, AHCPR convened a panel to set guidelines for the treatment of lower back pain. One of this panel's observations was that there was little evidence that widely used and expensive spinal fusion surgery was any better than other far less expensive, nonsurgical treatments. Surgeons who performed this procedure (and allies in the medical device business) saw this as a direct threat to a very lucrative surgical business and went directly to Congress. They created a firestorm that resulted in the budget for the *entire* AHCPR being eliminated in the House of Representatives. The organization was eventually saved, but with its budget considerably reduced and stripped of its authority to recommend *anything* to Medicare and Medicaid. Fifteen years later, we spend billions each year on spinal fusion surgery—$16 billion in 2004 and rising steeply—and there's still little evidence that it's better for anyone except the surgeons, the medical device manufacturers, and the hospitals. The panel needs the imprimatur of being created by Congress, but set up in a fashion that keeps it independent of political pressure through its budget after that.

In addition to its independence from budgetary pressure, the Standards Panel will be structured to remain as independent as possible of other interests, as well. Some of these other interests are also economic, and the panel's members should, of course, be free from conflicts arising from business interests, consulting contracts, and industry-sponsored research. Other interests are not strictly economic, but nevertheless strong, and they should be kept at arm's length as well. Various nonprofit organizations concentrate on specific diseases and naturally have strong feelings as to the importance of those diseases and the aggressiveness with which they should be diagnosed and treated. Various advocacy groups see the medical world in similar terms. Even professional associations representing various medical specialties, whose participation is needed, will have strong feelings about the importance of what their member physicians do. This isn't a criticism—we all believe in the importance of what we choose to do, that's why we do it. But it's a reality that the panel has to recognize and insulate itself from.

The panel will be charged with two tasks. First, to establish the standards of care that scientific evidence at any given time shows to be the best. Second, to establish a scoring mechanism that defines how to measure how well medical practice conforms to that standard.

Building a set of national practice standards will be difficult. We place a lot of faith today in the concept of evidence-based medicine as a vehicle to improve quality and the terms of our payment systems. The underlying science, however, on which we rely, is variable in its quality and spotty in its coverage. There are areas of consensus, where the research is good and there's broad agreement.

The proper treatment and management of diabetes would be a good example of such an area. For this diagnosis, there's excellent research and the American Diabetes Association has evaluated it carefully and published standards. Those standards are revised regularly and broadly accepted in the medical community. NCQA has adopted a set of standards for the treatment of both diabetes and a number of other common diagnoses and uses them to benchmark quality in America's health plans. These HEDIS measures, which we noted at the beginning of this chapter, are well-known and represent the broadest use today of objective quality measures. They provide a starting point for thinking about a comprehensive and robust system of standards.

However, while there are areas of excellence and consensus, there are also large areas of medicine where the research is limited or compromised and there are no accepted standards today. I asked a group of physicians recently for some examples of common patient problems where they felt they had little guidance from evidence-based medical standards. The first example, warmly seconded by all, was lower back pain.

In many cases, lower back pain is real, even if it can't be seen objectively, and the physician would like some help with the best protocols to address that patient's needs. The lack of standards here opens the door for surgical treatments that are expensive, not supported by independent evidence, and frequently harmful to the patient. Sometimes, back pain is faked: this is a common complaint brought to an emergency room for the purpose of securing narcotic prescriptions. One ER physician in this group told the story of a regular visitor who carried with him a spinal X-ray from the early nineties, carefully laminated to preserve it but dog-eared anyway. He'd present this as proof that he had intractable back pain, "as any idiot can see." In TennCare our record setter in 2005 was a young woman who visited twenty different hospital emergency rooms a total of 174 times. Clearly established standards would be very helpful here. Even if they're imperfect to begin, they would be an improvement on the inconsistent approaches that are used today. Standards would help guide and protect the doctors who saw this patient. They might also begin the process of pushing the health care system into dealing with her actual problem of drug addiction.

Similarly, a number of mental health diagnoses fall in this category. Bipolar disorders, for example, are widespread and debilitating, yet there's little consensus on their proper treatment. Mental health is a difficult area in which to conduct objective research. Nevertheless, these illnesses are now solidly (and properly) in the domain of medical care and rapidly approaching parity in the obligation to treat them. The establishment of standards in the area of mental health needs to move beyond reliance on self-serving pharmaceutical company research and become more independent and scientific.

The work of the Standards Panel would start simply and grow. It would begin with setting standards for the most common and important episodes of care where reliable research is available. Over the years it would continue to expand as research is evaluated and gaps filled in. It would most likely organize its work by diagnosis, with the concept of diagnosis extended to include preventive and well-care services in addition to actual illnesses. As a by-product of its work, the Standards Panel would identify those areas where expanded or better research is needed. That, in turn, would provide a guide for various organizations, both governmental and nongovernmental, in their funding of research.

In some areas, practice standards can be quite precise. Examples of these areas might include the proper treatment of a variety of chronic illnesses such as diabetes, asthma, emphysema, or coronary heart disease. Other areas might include appropriate prenatal care for mothers with various common risk factors and the proper preventive care for patients of various ages. In other areas, either the state of the science or the complexity of the disease may be such that more general standards are called for: the treatment of some cancers or trauma cases might fall in this category.

The product of this Standards Panel will always be a work in progress and we want it to be. Our understanding of diseases and treatments for them will evolve and improve over time, and we want to keep our standards up-to-date. Its underlying purpose however remains constant: to give structure and meaning to the idea of evidence-based medicine. It is charged to remain completely independent and professional, to look at the research, to evaluate its reliability and independence, and to distill from it what can be said at any given point about what is clinically best for the patient.

The limitations of evidence-based medicine

Like everything else, evidence-based medicine has its limitations. If we plan to give it a more central role in health care we should keep these limitations in mind. First, most of the research on which evidence-based medicine depends is conducted using the accepted gold standard in the medical field: randomized controlled trials to measure the effect of some treatment. Suppose a researcher wants to evaluate how well some proposed new drug controls blood pressure in people with red hair. To do that, she identifies a group of people with red hair who are willing to participate in a clinical trial. She gives some of them the drug and some of them a harmless and inert substitute—a placebo. The patients don't know which is which (and in the best trials neither does the researcher or her statistician). She measures every participant's blood pressure, and after a while the data on who got what pill is combined with the blood pressure data. What she's hoping to find is that those who took the real pill had some decline in their blood pressure and those who took the placebo didn't. This is the way in which she attempts to isolate the effects of her new drug from all the other things that might be going on affecting blood pressure.

The advantage of randomized controlled trials is that they're a sound and scientific yardstick for measuring things under controlled conditions. The disadvantage is that we humans are very complicated and messy beings; trying to cleanly isolate the effect the researcher is looking for can be very difficult. A drug might have completely unanticipated effects—both positive and negative—that aren't picked up in a randomized controlled trial because the researcher doesn't even know to look for them. Often effects don't make themselves known for a much longer period of time than any practical study could cover.

One shortcoming of a too-narrow reliance on evidence-based medicine shows up often when physicians deal with what are called comorbid conditions. This term describes the common situation in which a patient has more than one disease and the presence of each illness might affect and alter the decision-making process for treating the other. The doctor is confronted with a more complicated situation than "one disease in isolation and one right answer." An example of how easily evidence-based medicine can go wrong when things get complicated occurred just recently. It involved standards for the treatment of diabetes that worked for diabetes but were harmful when the patient also had heart disease—a common combination of conditions. In 2006, NCQA issued a diabetes treatment standard (which was being urged by the American Diabetes Association), which included aggressive control of blood sugar levels. The committee adopting the standard thought it a well-justified recommendation for patients with diabetes. However, physicians who followed this quality guideline with older patients who also had heart problems found their patients dying at unexpectedly high rates. The aggressive blood sugar control doubtless helped manage the diabetes, but it more than offset this benefit with what it did to the diseased hearts. The standard was promptly changed, but the lesson here is that things get complicated quickly where human biology is concerned. We need to recognize that the idealizations we incorporate in our standards are imperfect and can lead us astray, especially when dealing with complicated patients.

Another limitation of evidence-based medicine is that not all evidence is the same. Medicine is a very big business and it's an area where research is particularly vulnerable to economic pressures. There's a lot of university research funded by companies with large economic stakes in the outcomes and even fine researchers wouldn't be human not to feel some pressures as a result. More flagrantly, the *Journal of the American Medical Association* did a study in 2009 and reported that "six of the top medical journals published a significant number of articles in 2008 that were written by ghostwriters financed by drug companies." Those authors were engaging in the same behavior that gets college students thrown out of school, and we can safely assume that the ghostwriters were not paid by the drug companies to write scientifically objective research papers.

I believe it's important to acknowledge some of the limitations of evidence-based medicine. It's also important to keep this all in perspective. There is enormous scope to improve our health care system by setting practice standards and monitoring them. Once in a while, that approach will steer us wrong and we need to recognize that on-the-spot professional judgment is a safer course. But for every one of those there are a hundred times that good practice standards will improve the care that a patient receives.

Informed patients

While much of the measurement of quality will be about evidence-based medicine, there is another dimension to quality that we should incorporate as well. Patients, where appropriate, should be offered participation in decisions affecting them where the patient's own values become a part of the considerations. Good doctors try to do this, but out of respect for the patient we should elevate this to an integral part of the quality of medical care. It's something we should specify and then measure it right along with whether or not the right medicine is prescribed. A deep respect for each individual citizen and the right of that citizen to make her own decisions is a founding American value. We need to ensure that patients are allowed to be active participants in choices that affect them and not passive recipients of what the medical industry prescribes.

Today, the most common circumstance where this participation is called for is at the time of end-of-life decisions—how aggressively to treat terminal illnesses or whether to begin dialysis, for example. Unfortunately, this discussion seems to always takes place in a financial context—are we going to pay for your chemotherapy, or are you too old and sick? As long as we allow the patient to actually have the choice, I can't see any moral justification whatsoever in denying him information that might help make this choice. I recognize that this concept is at least a cousin to the more limited (and incompetently put forward) idea of end-of-life consultation that prompted the "death panel" charge. But politicians getting headlines pandering to people's fears doesn't do anything except to confirm them as charlatans. Denying citizens information they need to make intensely personal decisions under difficult circumstances is contemptible, not heroic.

Beyond these obvious situations, the number of options for medical treatment is becoming larger over time. There are a growing number of areas where the patient can be a participant in balancing various medical options against his or her own values. We began this chapter with the story of a woman who had been sold on the idea of a Cesarean section for the delivery of her baby. When a woman is delivering a baby and there are difficulties that threaten the health of either of them, the physician's job is to act decisively and competently. The patient's role is limited and she does what we all would do; she puts her trust in the skill and judgment of her physician.

On the other hand, we have a large and growing number of elective Cesarean sections performed in our country and in these

of quality in health care, that means setting down, diagnosis by diagnosis, just what should be measured, how that measurement should be taken, and its weight in the overall assessment of quality. This is the dashboard that we'll use to actually measure quality.

In the beginning, the Standards Panel's list of standards will be modest, and the Red Book will be correspondingly thin. As they start to fill in the blanks in standards and get experience and feedback, the book will grow. It doesn't contain the standards; that's more complex and appropriate as a communication from professional to professional. The Red Book will always be concise, with an emphasis on objective and numerical measurement; it will be a dashboard from which to read quality.

The best quality measurements are those that measure actual results. If a patient has high blood pressure, we want to give real weight in our quality measure to the actual outcome; to whether his blood pressure is actually controlled. If it is, we're less concerned about just what drug was used or exactly what kind of counseling was employed. Placing a premium on results puts more responsibility on the health care system to find an answer that works for that individual patient rather than just executing a script. Where we can, putting actual results first avoids the situation from the very old joke: "The operation was successful but the patient died."

In medicine, however, there are a lot of times where this doesn't work. Many of the outcomes we're seeking are a result of many factors, some of which are beyond the scope of medical care. If a patient has a heart attack, there's one obvious and important immediate result: does he survive the heart attack or not? The care he receives in the emergency room is definitely a factor in that, but there are many others as well. Heart attacks come in very different levels of severity. Some patients arrive at the hospital quickly, some more slowly. Patients have different ages, overall health, and genetics. Here we're on safer ground measuring whether the medical care, once he arrives at the hospital, adheres to the standards we've developed.

Moreover, many of the results we care about happen sometime in the future. Even if we can isolate them from other factors, as a practical matter we need working measures that are available quickly and can be used as feedback to manage our health care system. If a physician is treating a patient with diabetes, a large part of what she's doing is minimizing the long-term effects of the disease. But it does us no good to have to wait twenty years to be able to measure the quality of the care the doctor provided by waiting to see the outcome for that patient. That's an important role for research—looking at the long-term consequences of decisions. But for practical use, we then translate that into a set of standards for the treatments that the physician should use right now. We measure quality against that process rather than the final results.

Measuring quality: diabetes

The easiest way to explain the approach that I'm proposing is to take a specific example and see what it might look like. I've picked a common, growing, and expensive diagnosis: diabetes mellitus (uncomplicated). As we discussed earlier in this chapter, this is a diagnosis for which there's already considerable consensus on what constitutes excellent care. I'm obviously not a physician who can professionally defend the individual items, but I've discussed this in considerable depth with those who are and believe this is a practical example.

Table 4 represents what the entry in the Red Book dealing with this diagnosis might look like. You'll notice that it assigns a total of one hundred quality points that can theoretically be achieved. It then breaks that total down into several subsections with their own scores. The evaluation of the management of HbA1C levels represents 20 points, for example. (For the nonmedical reader, HbA1C is a laboratory test performed on blood cells that averages blood

Table 4
Quality Dashboard for Diabetes mellitus (uncomplicated)

ICD-9	250	Diabetes mellitus (uncomplicated)	
Total Points		Item	Time Period (months)
20		HbA1C Levels Checked	12
		< 7% (20)	
		< 9% (16)	
		>9%	
		Appropriate Rx (5)	
		Independent monitor of Rx compliance (2)	
		Patient consult/contact 2x (5)	
20		**Blood Pressure Checked**	12
		<130/80 (20)	
		<140/90 (16)	
		>140/90	
		Appropriate Rx (5)	
		Independent monitor of Rx compliance (2)	
		Patient consult/contact 2x (5)	
20		**LDL-C Screen**	12
		<100 (20)	
		<140 (16)	
		>140	
		Appropriate Rx (5)	
		Independent monitor of Rx compliance (2)	
		Patient consult/contact 2x (5)	
15		**Aspirin Considered/Prescribed**	12
10		**Foot Exam Performed**	12
10		**Eye Exam Performed**	12
5		**Appropriate take-with care instructions provided**	12
100			

Modifiers:

1   Items performed more than twelve months but less than 24 score at .75 x basic score

2   If patient not seen twelve months, 60 points for 2x attempts to schedule in past twelve months

sugar levels over time, the LDL-C Screen is a blood cholesterol measurement, the eye and foot exams are to look for early signs of damage from the disease that might later result in blindness or amputation; the rest of the measures should be self-explanatory.)

One aspect that is immediately noticeable is how specific the diabetes mellitus dashboard is. It sets out goals that are unambiguous and that can be scored by looking at patient charts. The goal is to have as many measures as possible that don't require judgment to score. As time goes on, we'll want most of this scoring done by information systems that review electronic patient records, with humans reserved for the exceptions. While the numerical targets that I've used in this example would be broadly supported, as with anything in medicine, there is still debate and they will likely evolve over time. For example, awarding the highest number of points to the control of HbA1C levels under 7% is considered by some professionals to be too aggressive (and we earlier discussed the problem with this in patients who also have heart disease). We are, however, asking the panel to make a call here, to set a level, to specify exceptions, and then to modify the dashboard from time to time as further research is available.

Most of the scoring is not a yes/no checklist, but considers levels of performance. For example, with regard to HbA1C levels, the full score (20 points) is assigned to levels under 7%, but almost the full score (16 points) to levels under 9%. A similar approach is taken with blood pressure and with the cholesterol screen. For those patients where the desired levels are not reached (where the HbA1C is over 9%, for example) we then look at the underlying process. In that case, there are points for prescribing an appropriate medicine, points for independently checking on compliance (for example, if the prescriptions are being filled), and points for contacting or counseling the patient at least twice in the preceding twelve months. This recognizes that there are circumstances where the disease is simply more difficult to control, and often circumstances where patients refuse to comply. In these cases we want to reward the correct effort.

However, running through this scoring process is a preference for results: actually getting the HbA1C or LDL-C or blood pressures to the desired levels is always more valuable than just trying. We always want the medical care system to be seeking ways to achieve the desired results; doing the best we know how is always a little more valuable than getting the result. Notice also that when the desired results are achieved, we don't score the process; if the HbA1C level is satisfactory, we don't question the prescription or require consultation; the results speak for themselves.

The concept of "appropriate Rx" doesn't include trade-offs of costs and benefits. It's simply whether a prescription appropriate to the patient's condition has been written. The provider group will have its own standards designed to control costs while keeping quality high. It may, for example, call for trying a frequently successful and less expensive drug such as metformin first. In many patients that drug will work with complete success. If it doesn't, then the physician moves on to other options, such as more expensive brand formulations or combinations. But we don't muddy our quality measure by mixing it at the front end with cost considerations; quality is always simply about what our research has found to be most effective.

Some other items in our entry are simple yes/no items. The consideration of aspirin, the eye and foot exam, the take-away instructions. Remember that this is a dashboard. We'll assume that the professional is competent to perform the exams and simply want to know if they have been completed. As time goes on, we'll undoubtedly want to further refine these. The idea of "appropriate" take-with care instructions might be refined to include the availability of materials that are appropriate to someone who doesn't read or doesn't read English. It might ultimately reward sophisticated educational materials much more highly that a copied typewritten sheet. As experts consider these dashboard measures, it might also be appropriate at some point to incorporate measures of improvement for difficult patients, to reward progress toward the established goals.

This dashboard is designed to be about the care that a specific patient receives: What is the score for patient X? It's not a measure of the percentage of the time that these standards are met in a practice or in a health plan. It's also designed to be tough enough that few perfect scores are given. The goal is to set up a tension where medical care is trying to maximize the quality scores they can achieve with the constraints of limited resources. To do that, there always needs to be room for further improvement.

Cookbook medicine

As we work to put more structure around the practice of medicine by defining standards of care and ways of measuring quality, one obvious objection would be that doing so installs "cookbook medicine" in America. No one wants such a thing, and highly trained physicians and other medical professionals need great discretion in their treatment decisions, especially in complex cases. Any evaluation of quality has to provide clear and broad paths for exceptions when the physician feels a different path to be in the best interest of her patient and we'll discuss the mechanics of how the Red Book would be used in the next chapter.

It's an inescapable fact that medical care in America is far more varied in how it's practiced than is justified by the underlying science. The huge regional variations in care, by themselves, are proof of this. Some of the variation results from the considered professional judgment of the physician and we need always to protect that option. Much of it, however, is rooted in habit, in a lack of knowledge, or in economic considerations. It's reasonable to ask that when a physician deviates from clear and accepted scientific standards she at least knows what those standards are and has responsible reasons for the deviation. When she does, we'll defer to her.

This has brought us now to our fourth stepping-stone—quality. We've begun the process of bringing modern quality assurance tools to the practice of medicine. Our first step has been to establish a system of standards for the practice of medicine and a way to measure medical care against them. This is the tool we'll use to develop our quality metric, and in the next chapter we'll put it to use in a specific way.

10

Stepping-Stone Five: Systems of Care

... in which we introduce a large change that we propose to make to American health care—rebuilding its basic structure around systems of care. We'll define these as organizations that are paid a fixed annual amount for each of their members, have considerable flexibility in their operation, and are responsible for both delivering medical care to their members and for measuring the quality of that care.

Up to this point, I've been pulling things apart, trying to strip away the extraneous and find the simple things that count. We explored why the insurance paradigm that permeates the health care system is obsolete. We looked at values that might guide us and I've proposed three core ones: access to medical care with dignity and privacy, the equitable treatment of Americans who are in similar situations, and universal care. We saw that we incorporated similar values seventy-five years ago in a highly successful social insurance program called Social Security. We saw that the underlying problem in the cost of health care was that we had systematically eliminated the economic tension between buyers and sellers that makes the marketplace work.

We looked at the organization of American health care, and I argued that it was too large, loosely connected, and dominated by powerful local incentives to be responsive to traditional top-down management. I called this characteristic "hypercomplexity" and attempted to show that it can be managed most successfully through establishing a three-step cycle—innovation, measurement, and selection—that operates in an environment of limited resources. I proposed that the problem with applying this concept to the management of our health care system was the lack of a suitable measurement for the second step—a way of objectively grading what was good and bad in any particular episode of care. We discussed how we could construct an artificial measurement using the concepts of evidence-based medicine.

We've been assembling a lot of building blocks. Now it's time to synthesize—to take our building blocks and put them together in a new configuration. This new way to organize the delivery of our health care is our fifth stepping-stone—systems of care.

A better way to deliver health care

We have some tools now, but we need a place to put them to work. We've already seen that it's difficult to do so at the level of individual patients. We patients don't have the expertise to evaluate medical quality. We're inevitably at a distance from the economics where expensive care is concerned. We're often involved in an extremely emotional fashion that clouds our thinking. The concept of patient-*centered* care is a powerful one, but the concept of patient-*managed* care doesn't work. We've also seen that trying to establish incentives at the level of physician groups or hospitals has many problems and unintended consequences as well. More important, it still fails to address the overall coordination and intelligent resource allocation that is needed so badly in medicine. Either one still leaves medicine in the fragmented mess that it's in now. Yet, at the other organizational extreme, top down doesn't work either. Health care is just too big and complex.

Instead, we need to apply our incentives at a level in our health care system that's right-sized. It has to be big enough to bring together all the threads of care for any individual—primary care, specialty care, outpatient services, drugs, hospitals, and so on—in one place where they can be balanced and coordinated. It also needs to be small enough that it's manageable internally with traditional management techniques.

The way to accomplish this is to build our health care system around what I'm calling "systems of care." The concept is an old one, and what I mean specifically by this phrase is a formal organization that receives a determined payment for each of its patients, takes responsibility for the delivery, quality, coordination, and payment for health care for those who belong to it, and which competes with other systems of care in its geographic area for the business of citizens. Each of those citizens selects the system of care they prefer, and then receives their health care through that system. The systems of care have considerable latitude to innovate, the quality of care they provide is carefully audited and made very public, and they live or die, grow or decline based on their ability to compete. Systems of care are the vehicle to finally leave behind the outdated and counterproductive insurance model for health care.

The phrase "system of care" is already a familiar one in the health care world. It's most commonly used to describe a coordinated approach to providing services to children and it's also used in the same sense for mental health services. What I'm doing is applying the concept to medical care in general, and adding some additional elements to it as well. A system of care in this approach is a formally organized and comprehensive medical care organization, not a loose collection of doctors and hospitals. It could be non-profit or for-profit, it could be a cooperative, it could even be a unit of government itself. Many of the institutions that are already involved in the delivery of health care—Blue Cross or a large hospital, for example—are already a rudimentary form of our system of care. They will have three responsibilities, two of which will be immediately familiar and one which will not.

First, a system of care has *financial responsibility* for the medical care of each person belonging to it. We're going to give it a fixed annual payment (it will depend on age and sex, of course) for each member, and then it's responsible for all the medical care for that member. Fixing the total amount is key—in order to put our three-step process to work, we need to be operating in an environment of limited resources. This is a familiar concept—any insurance company or managed care organization does this. Any company or union health care trust fund does as well. The difference is that we're going to tie these amounts directly to the taxes that individuals experience, so that there's real pressure to contain them and not just pass them on.

We've already noted that while any insurance company will have various cost containment measures in place they're still insurance companies. They have little direct control over the delivery system and their basic business remains a financial one. They try to accurately predict future costs, set premium rates sufficient to cover them, and pay the claims that come in. Even managed care organizations that combine aspects of payment and care delivery do so in a comfortable environment where the costs of their competitors grow rapidly and provide them with a generous cost umbrella. For those organizations that assume financial responsibility today, managing those costs is a modest side dish, not the main course. With the new systems of care, that's no longer the case. They're operating entities, not financial intermediaries. There's no comfortable and steadily growing umbrella.

Our plan for managing hypercomplexity starts with creating a world of limited resources in which these systems of care compete for a place. We'll constrain the resources in each system by setting the payment levels and tying them directly to the trust fund we're going to create. We're not setting levels of payments or rates of increase in advance, only committing to keeping the trust fund solvent. We can always adjust, but increasing payments to the systems of care more than the trust fund revenues grow will require a tax increase. This payment mechanism will be national in scope and, after an adjustment period, essentially the same everywhere. It will work because there's nowhere else to go—these payments made for each member is the way that basic health care gets paid for in America. In that environment, for a system of care to be successful it will have to bring to bear all the tools that management science has to offer. It will have to innovate and negotiate because it's in a competitive environment and if it fails to do so, someone else will. It will always be under pressure from the system down the road. It actually can fail, go out of business, and watch a competitor pick up its patients. No one can predict what the health care issues will be in ten, twenty, or thirty years, but whatever they are, competition with real consequences will ensure that every system will address them as effectively as they can.

The second responsibility of a system of care is also familiar to us: it *provides medical care*. There are organizations in our health care system today that do exactly that. A large, tightly integrated health maintenance organization such as Kaiser Permanente assumes responsibility for and directly provides most of the care for its 8.6 million members, with a budget of $40 billion (2008). The Veterans Health Administration system does the same for a large number of service veterans.

Even more conventional parts of our health care system such as insurance companies, although they're at heart financial institutions, already assume some responsibility in this regard. They have some choices in deciding which providers of medical care to contract with. They frequently impose administrative mechanisms to approve drugs or medical procedures before they'll pay for them. While these are first of all measures to help manage costs, they have an impact on how medical care is delivered and therefore assume a role in managing its delivery. Many insurance companies also contract with organizations that provide disease management services for chronic illnesses such as diabetes. Those arrangements also represent a direct involvement in the delivery of that care.

There are conventional fee-for-service medical providers whose comprehensive approach is close to what we're seeking. A large university hospital with its associated outpatient services and faculty practice can be almost a self-contained system of care in its own right. Community hospitals that have built large associated physician practices have some of this characteristic as well, although typically without the degree of integration that an academic medical center achieves. Specialized organizations such as the Mayo Clinic are perhaps the most tightly integrated providers of comprehensive medical services that we have in our country today.

Today, good health care is organized health care, and building medical care around organized systems of care will improve it in many ways. The number of elderly, for example, is going to continue to increase, and more patients with medical issues that are multi-dimensional will require coordinated treatment. My mother was quite ill a few years ago, and saw several specialists during that time, all of whom had practices located on the campus of the same community hospital. They didn't coordinate her care, frequently told her conflicting things, and occasionally one would countermand the orders written by another. This is not a complaint about the qualifications of those specialists, which to the best of my knowledge were individually excellent. It's rather about the clear need for organizational changes that would allow their efforts to be better coordinated.

The practice of medicine is beginning to return to an ethic in which the highest quality health care involves treating each patient as a whole. We're starting to move beyond seeing each person as a vessel for compartmentalized problems to be identified and treated separately. As the years go by, the need to integrate and coordinate medical care will only continue to grow. Systems of care can take us there.

The third responsibility, however, is new. Our systems of care will also have complete and final *responsibility for the quality of medical care* that they provide. Of course, any provider already has responsibility for the quality of care it provides. We're bumping the final responsibility up a level, to the organization that is coordinating and financing that care. We'll carefully and comprehensively measure the quality of care that they organize. That's the measurement that will judge a system of care's performance and put our three-step cycle to work.

For this to work, the systems will need considerably more freedom to innovate and make changes than we now allow. We won't set rates for services as we now do with Medicare and parts of Medicaid. They'd make no sense anyway as the systems will need to depart from the traditional fee-for-service payment method in order to compete. We'll have to preempt state laws that protect various economic interests. The structure in which systems of care operate will have rules, but ones designed only to establish base requirements in areas such as licensing, financial soundness, adequacy of their medical delivery system, and accuracy and clarity in their marketing claims.

Now we have our basic building block for health care—the system of care. There will likely be hundreds of them, and each will operate in a world of limited resources. Each will have latitude to innovate and will have to do so to compete effectively. Each has responsibility for the quality of care they provide and that quality will be carefully measured and reported. Each will compete openly for the business of citizens who are free to choose. Those who provide quality and keep costs down will prosper, those that don't will decline or go out of business. And that's exactly the approach we've identified for managing hypercomplexity: limited resources, innovation, measurement, selection.

National Independent Quality Audit

Every time we find high quality in goods or services, we almost always find the organizations involved in producing them have taken quality seriously. They've taken the time to decide just what quality is, they've embedded it as an integral part of creating the goods, and they've often set up a way to independently check on just how well these mechanisms are working. Quality becomes a part of the culture of the organization. In the last chapter, I described a starting point with national practice standards and a dashboard for measuring care against them. Now let's see how to use this framework to measure quality for our systems of care.

The way to accomplish this in health care is to set up a formal, well-funded, and nationally sanctioned auditing process. This can't be a government review, which would be subject to political considerations, and most likely not trusted by the public. Rather, it will be an independent process that builds on the unbiased and professional approach that we used to construct practice standards and the Red Book.

I'm envisioning a comprehensive effort at an entirely different level of commitment than we currently employ. It would seem reasonable, for example, to commit one quarter of 1% of our health care expenditures to actually measure and check on how well the medical care system is delivering care. If I visit my doctor and he performs (and my employer and I pay for) $500 worth of work, it seems completely sensible to me to spend $1.25 of that to expertly and independently verify the correctness of what I'm getting. Taken to a national level, even that modest commitment would pay for an effort vastly more sophisticated and comprehensive than anything that's done today. Nationally, in 2011, it would amount to about $6.8 billion of auditing. To put that in more comprehensible terms, in Tennessee it would translate to a quality audit effort funded annually at about $135 million; in Florida, $400 million; in South Dakota, $18 million.

In order to accomplish this review, we'd start by establishing a series of quality audit centers around the country. There would be an umbrella organization, independent of government, which would be charged with the designation and commissioning of these audit organizations and the ongoing review of their performance. The National Committee for Quality Assurance (NCQA) might serve well in this role. They've been committed for a long time to measuring and reporting the quality of medical care and an undertaking such as this would build nicely on the mission and expertise of the organization.

They (or another organization) would then create a number of quality audit centers. There would be enough of these to keep them individually at a manageable size, and few enough to allow each of them the critical mass of resources they would need to be stable and successful. Roughly speaking, twenty of these with a thousand employees each would fit within the budget. That seems like a stunning number on first glance: twenty buildings, each managing a thousand employees and housing extensive computer systems—the federal government once again run wild. It only seems that way because of the vast size of our health care system. It represents about two weeks of *inflation* today.

We'd want some diversity in how these centers are organized, but attaching some of them to existing medical care organizations would have many benefits. A connection of some with academic medical centers could be particularly advantageous, both for the expertise it would make available to the centers and the opportunity for training medical care professionals it would provide to the institutions.

As we'll see, in auditing quality of care, there will be many situations where a judgment will need to be made by a physician or other expert. This physician involvement is an opportunity to involve practicing physicians in the audits as well. This involvement provides a real-world component to the review and will keep the process anchored to reality. It will also generate invaluable feedback to the Standards Panel and the Red Book. Perhaps most important, it can also be a powerful force to establish the culture of evidence-based quality in our health care system. I can imagine a world in a couple of decades where any physician, as an integral part of her professional ethic and responsibility, devotes a couple of days each year to participating in quality audits.

The audit would begin with staff members of the audit centers going to provider locations and sampling the contents of selected medical records. The records to be selected would be based on the relative importance assigned to various types of episodes of care and the statistical considerations of getting reliable samples. Where the records are in paper form, the information is assembled manually. Where there are electronic medical records being used it will clearly go more smoothly and efficiently. The job would be to identify the records, abstract the information in them in a standard form, and then make them anonymous as to both the patient and provider. Patient anonymity is obviously needed for privacy and provider anonymity guarantees that the records to be audited are not colored by the reputation of the provider or the concept of "community standards." These records are then distributed to the audit bodies on a random basis so that inevitable variations in approach (and toughness) among the audit centers would be evened out.

The result of this process would be a continuous flow of standardized abstracts of various episodes of care to the audit centers. They would be anonymous to the centers receiving them, and randomly distributed around the country. A medical group in New York would expect to have some of its own records that had been selected for audit being examined in every one of the audit centers. Similarly, any given audit center would be examining records from providers across the nation. We'd doubtless inject some created test records into the stream to check, in turn, on the consistency and accuracy of the process at the various audit centers—we'd audit the auditors.

Each audit center would then process these abstracts in several different ways. First, many of them will be straightforward and the audits likely to be automated: I'll call these the basic records. When we were considering the specific example of uncomplicated diabetes and the Red Book entry that would represent it, we described items that can be straightforwardly measured and for which little or no judgment is required. Much of the work that NCQA does today is in this category: given a diagnosis, what are the values of a few key parameters and did certain things called for by evidence-based medical standards happen or not? What's the patient's blood pressure? Did the eye exam take place or not? This part of the audit would likely be highly automated.

There is a second class of records that would be handled differently: I'll call these the professional exception records. We want to ensure that physicians and other health care professionals always have the freedom to exercise their judgment. A physician's first responsibility is to the patient. There will be times when she believes that some alternative course of action other than what is called for by the standard is in their patient's best interest. We should give that judgment great deference, just as we do with other highly trained professionals such as airline pilots or military commanders. We've already seen that for patients with diabetes. The recommended standard a few years ago for how aggressively to treat patients to lower their blood sugar was wrong and actually harmful to patients who also had heart disease. There were many physicians who believed the recommended practice to be wrong and ignored it; their patients benefited from this exercise of professional judgment.

The quality audit for these professional exception records would defer to a notation by the physician that she had chosen an alternative course. Perhaps in our diabetes example, she would make a notation of "HbA1c of 7.0 too aggressive, elderly, heart disease." We're not asking for an elaborate justification of her decision— she doesn't have to quote medical journal articles—but simply an indication that she knows what the standard is, has considered it before selecting a different course of treatment, and has indicated her line of thinking. If the reason she states is within the bounds of reasonable professional discretion then the audit of that record would give deference to that professional call.

There is, of course, the potential for abuse here—one can envision a physician trying to improve scores by just noting in every diabetic's record "7.0 too aggressive." That can be controlled by requiring an indication of the rationale, the "elderly, heart disease" notation, which can be checked and verified if necessary. With these professional exception records, audit centers would use medical professionals to design approaches to handling situations and set parameters as to what represents generous but scientifically responsible professional variation. As these exceptions are accumulated in the audits, patterns will emerge of those areas where professional exceptions are frequently taken. This feedback will allow the Standards Panel to control abuse, to reconsider the standards they have adopted, and to expand standards to accommodate common exceptions. It will also allow them to recommend further research in an area where there is widespread professional disagreement.

The third class of records are those that reflect especially complex episodes of care, or medical care related to diagnoses where there have not been evidence-based standards developed. These would be reviewed and scored by a small panel of experts who would review the record with their own professional judgment of what would be appropriate in the circumstances. As before, the reviewers would approach this with deference to the decisions made by the provider so long as they represented a defensible professional approach. In order to efficiently perform these audit reviews for complex records, the audit center staff would organize the information and prepare summaries, highlighting any areas that might especially warrant review. After this preparation, the review would then take place by a panel of physicians with suitable expertise.

The end result of all this activity will be a large and growing collection of records of individual episodes of care. Each record contains the details of how that specific episode was handled together with a scoring that measures how well that treatment conforms to evidence-based professional standards. This collection of information, on its own, will offer an unprecedented window into the world of health care in America. The mere fact of its existence will focus the attention of providers on quality standards and itself improve quality. This body of information will also become a powerful research tool. Data mining such a vast and standardized database could be used to improve the practice standards themselves and identify problems with treatments or drugs quickly. It will be an early warning system for public health—how much earlier and more clearly might the HIV crisis have been identified with such an audit in place? By identifying the most widespread weaknesses, it will improve health care professional training and continuing education. However, the best is yet to come.

The final step

Despite all the obvious benefits of such a comprehensive audit, the real purpose is to set up the metric that defines what we want our systems of care to do. So, as our final step, we'll reunite all these individual scores with the system in which they originated, roll them up, and use them to assign a single numerical quality score to every system of care in the country. Blue Cross of Western Pennsylvania, 82; the East Tennessee Rural Health Cooperative, 79; the Vanderbilt University Hospital and Faculty Practice Plan, 89; Kaiser Permanente Oregon, 87. We'll publicize these widely and require that advertising and marketing communications from the systems feature the scores prominently.

Systems of care will be forced to compete for the business of each American in their service area. In making her choice, each American will have at hand an understandable and objective measure of the quality of care that the system is providing. That determination is not made by government, nor by a magazine, nor by anyone with a financial interest in the provision of that care. It's based on the standards set by physicians, measured by an independent auditor against those standards, and reported directly to her in a fashion she can use in making her choice.

In order to do this, the various episodes that have been scored by the audit centers have to be weighted by their frequency of occurrence and the health implications of correct treatment. The relative importance of quality scores for the treatment of asthma would be greater than for the treatment of malaria because asthma is far more common. Similarly, the weight assigned to the correct treatment of heart attacks is greater than that assigned to correctly treating a common cold because of the greater health impact of getting it right where heart attacks are concerned.

These weightings don't need to be static, and changing them in an orderly way will be a simple and powerful tool to shift the focus of the entire health care system in response to new challenges.

While we all dread the prospect, as the years go by there will be other challenges like that presented by AIDS. Imagine if in the late 1980s there had been a Red Book and an independent quality audit. That combination would have been a powerful tool to identify the problem. It would have had even greater value as a way to rapidly combat the spread of the epidemic. The standards of care in the Red Book relating to routine preventive care could have been quickly altered to give considerable weight to HIV testing and patient education in at-risk populations. The weights assigned to those scores could have been increased to give them more importance. This would have given our nation the lever to bring our mainstream health care system quickly into the fight. Archimedes claimed that if he had a lever and a place to stand, he could move the Earth. With a set of standards and comprehensive quality audits in place, the Red Book becomes a lever that can, with the effort of a pen stroke, move American health care.

Of course, people aren't going to base their entire decision about joining a system of care solely on a quality number. I might well choose a system of care that scores lower than another choice based on other considerations that are important to me. Convenience and access would certainly enter into it. I had a personal physician I trusted but who was a member of a lower-scoring system of care, I might well decide to remain with her and trust her to ensure that my own care was superior. Special competence in some area that interests me might be a factor as well.

But there's little question that the quality number assigned to a system would be an extremely powerful competitive factor. It's safe to assume that our systems would work hard to ensure high ratings and avoid low ones. Once a system actually takes responsibility for the quality of the care it's delivering, its outlook and priorities will change. It now has a strong reason to invest in clinical and patient information systems to monitor care. It has a strong reason to educate and assist providers in improving what they do. A system will prefer physicians and hospitals that can improve their scores and will avoid those that detract from them. That in turn will provide strong economic and professional incentives for providers to pay attention to quality and put in place their own systems to monitor and improve it.

The immediate and obvious objection to assigning simple quality scores to systems of care will be that "quality" is far too complex to reduce to a single dimension. But if you'll reflect back on our discussion of hypercomplexity, we observed that very simplicity is *exactly* what makes successful complex systems like market economies or natural selection work. They both embody a metric—the price of some product or the number of successful offspring produced—that integrates a large number of effects that are hard to compare into a single measurement.

We can (and do) discuss at length whether a system of care should invest in more family practitioners or a better health records system. I could make a good case for either one. It's a complicated choice with a lot of factors, obvious and not so obvious, that bear on it. The solution is to let economics and competition go to work. Let the systems try what they think is best and *measure the outcome*—the quality of care in the way we've defined it. The mix of strategies to improve care would likely be quite different among different providers and different medical cultures around the nation. The entire decision-making process about how resources are allocated in health care would no longer set by Congress or HHS, it would be about finding out, situation by situation, what actually works.

Health information systems

I started working in the health care field in the 1970s, applying information system technology to health care. I'm still at it today, and in Tennessee we've invested public funds and had some real success using regional health information organizations (RHIOs) to facilitate the interchange of medical information. Yet, of all the signs that there are fundamental problems with the organization of our health care system, the one that is clearest and most telling to me is its failure to make wide use of information technology. Health care is at its heart an information business, and yet, outside of hospitals and a few large organizations such as Kaiser Permanente or the Mayo Clinic, medical care has been very resistant.

Something is clearly wrong here. We're having to push this technology out into health care with grants, incentives, and laws. There's little pull from the health care system itself. In other parts of our economy, successful organizations invest in information technology to reduce costs and improve their product. Organizations from small businesses to Fortune 500 companies use it to make themselves more successful, and they certainly don't wait for government grants, let alone financial incentives from their customers, to do so. I'm confident that Boeing uses computers extensively in every aspect of designing and building their airplanes. It doesn't take special incentives to get their engineers to abandon their graph paper for computer screens.

The reason for the difference between Boeing and a group of doctors is straightforward: to Boeing, it matters and to the average Dr. Jones, it doesn't. Boeing operates in a world of normal economics and competes. If it doesn't use every tool at its command to produce well-designed airplanes at competitive prices, it can be assured that Airbus will, and Boeing will go out of business. Dr. Jones operates in a very different world. If she repeats some tests because she doesn't have the results that were obtained elsewhere it doesn't really matter—the cost of the repeated tests is passed on invisibly. If the patient doesn't get optimal care because information from other parts of the health care system is missing, it's likely that no one even notices.

Systems of care, operating in a competitive environment with limited resources, will completely change this picture. They'll invest in information technology, not because they're exhorted to do so or offered temporary financial incentives, but in order to compete effectively in a world where there are winners and losers. Winners will have made those investments; losers will have failed to.

Natural selection and the way in which it pushes life to adapt and succeed is inherent and natural. A market economy is more of a hybrid: its institutions are man-made, but the millions of individual trades of one thing for another that make it work are wired into the way we act as social animals. Managing our sprawling health care system to efficiently give us what we want and continuously adapt to change requires an even more "man-made" approach. The institution I've proposed we build—the system of care—is an existing and obvious idea. But inventing a metric in the form of a quality measurement to steer its behavior is an artifice unlike the more natural metrics of selection or market economies.

But this is what we need to do to take control. Very large, important, but loosely organized systems, such as our nation's health care, are a new feature of modern society. The capabilities of medical care will continue to grow exponentially and our society has long since accepted the responsibility of providing access to these capabilities. This is a challenge that neither our ancient genes nor the organizations of our industrial age are up to. Flogging away with more of the same won't work; the problem calls for us to step back and look at things differently.

We travel the world quickly and safely today. This isn't because we've used our wealth to assemble ever larger teams of horses and feed them ever growing helpings of oats. We do so because we took the time to understand how nature works and—after lots of false starts—used that understanding to figure out how to build jet engines and radios and airplane wings. We approached travel from a different direction.

In this past century, science has provided medicine with new and more powerful tools. What we haven't figured out yet is how to best assemble these tools into an efficient and effective health care system. When we do figure this out, the answer won't be to push ahead with ever larger teams of horses. It won't be to use our wealth to further fatten what we're already doing, hiring even more people, and buying even more pills. The answer will come from understanding better how our sprawling, hypercomplex health care system works and then using that new knowledge to bend it to our purposes.

So we arrive at our fifth stepping-stone: the organization of our health care system around multiple systems of care. These systems have limited resources, competing for the business of our citizens, and constantly making small adjustments to move steadily toward the best care that can be provided with the resources we've committed.

11

Stepping-Stone Six:
Paying for Health Care

... in which we find a better way to pay for health care.
We commit to paying in full for the health care we consume,
we establish a trust fund and fund it with a modern analog
of the Social Security payroll tax. We then give each
American a voucher with which to purchase a basic level
of health care—the "standard plan"—from whatever system
of care they wish. Individuals, organizations, and state
and local government are all free to add additional
services as they desire.

Let me warn you, at the outset of this chapter, that you won't find
in the pages to come any scheme to tweak how we pay for health
care in America. We've just been through one with the Affordable
Care Act, where we did all our work on the margins of health care.
Congress increased a couple of taxes, listed some planned savings,
and used the resulting financial headroom to buy or assist in buying health insurance for thirty-four million Americans. The underlying structure and finances of health care were left largely alone.
This is like thinking that the waves on the surface are all there is
to the ocean.

I'm approaching this issue from an entirely different direction: that the way we're paying for health care now is unsustainable and has generally become a baroque and unfair mess. It doesn't need tweaking; it needs replacing. That replacement, however we ultimately decide to go about it, has to start with the principle that we're actually going to *pay* for our health care and not pass the responsibility off to another generation.

Being honest about money

Like most Americans, I can easily understand the need to borrow during emergencies, such as wars or to smooth the effects of downturns in our economy. I supported the president's stimulus package for just that reason. But I can't think of a single reason why it's appropriate to borrow from anyone, let alone China, to pay the day-to-day costs of going to the doctor, getting a prescription filled, or spending time in the hospital. Nor can I think of a single reason why we should have any right to pass these costs on to our children and grandchildren. As you'll see, what it takes to actually pay for all we've decided we want is sobering but something that has to be faced. We should start paying our health care bills in America, in full, when they're due. When we face what that actually means, we may also get more serious about just what we're willing to pay for.

One good way to start is by laying on the table in front of us just how much we pay for health care and where the money is coming from. Right now, we obfuscate what we're doing with tax dollars and borrowings flowing through a myriad of little braided channels. We've already discussed at some length the importance of creating economic tension in health care transactions. The value of that principle isn't limited solely to purchasing individual medical services. Having some of that tension in our national health care considerations would be valuable as well.

The public debates about what medical care is guaranteed as a right and what limitations we're willing to place on it take on a different and healthier tone when the costs of those choices are clear and can be directly felt by every American. The tension someone feels when they decide how much they want to spend on a car—what features they need and what competing priorities they have—works just fine when we consider health care policy at the national level as well. The years ahead are likely to offer a lot of these choices. There are already cancer treatments that quickly run into the hundreds of thousands of dollars for modest and uncertain results. I've no doubt that our future holds artificial organs and other miracles that will comfortably surpass even these in their cost. Politicians may and will fulminate at length against "rationing," but the day is rapidly coming when, say, a third of all Americans can extend their lives for a couple of years with treatments that cost a large fraction of their lifetime earnings. When that happens, we start running out of other people to pay for what we want. We have some choices to make. Political leaders need to trust Americans—we as a people are perfectly capable of making very difficult choices *if* we can see and feel, not only the benefits, but also the costs. We do it all the time. When Americans are presented with these choices in a clear way, they will likely become the most powerful force we have for containing costs.

Let's do another thought experiment. Imagine an employee who earns $18 an hour in a factory job—an annual salary of $36,000—and has generous family health insurance as a benefit from her employer. This insurance has all manner of first dollar coverage and extra benefits and she loves it. Her employer's share of this insurance is $14,000 annually. Now this employer offers her (and all her coworkers) the following deal: "we're going to raise your wages from $16 an hour to $25 an hour; from $36,000 a year to $50,000. That's a 39% pay increase. Our cost of employing you doesn't change at all because we're going to eliminate our share of the cost of your health benefit.

"We've given you that raise and it's in your pocket. Now you have two options. We'll still offer you exactly the health insurance you have now—you give back that wage increase and go back to $18 an hour and we'll continue applying that $14,000 to your health insurance. Everything will be back to exactly where it is now. However, as an alternative, we have a less expensive health insurance plan that you can select and it will cost you $7,000 a year. It provides a safety net if one of your family members has a real problem, but for a lot of the routine care you'll have to pay a substantial share and there are some discretionary things it doesn't cover. If you choose that, you'll pay for it with $7,000 of your new raise and can keep the other $7,000 for yourself—a 19½% raise.

Is there anyone who doubts for a moment that large numbers of these employees with their $36,000 annual wage will choose a less comprehensive plan that puts almost 20% more cash in their pocket? The free checkups are very nice in isolation. But when there's the alternative of using the money they cost to purchase something for a child or their home that they can't afford now, that last bit of health care won't seem so attractive in comparison. This thought experiment just reminds us of the obvious. We want all the "free" things we can get. When we have to pay for something, and in doing so forego other things we want as well, we're willing to compromise and we start to make smart choices that reflect our values.

What part of our national wealth we dedicate to health care is ultimately our choice and will reflect what we value in our lives. There's no right number for how much we should devote to health care. It could be 10%, or 20%, or for that matter 30% of our gross national product, depending on how highly we value health care relative to the other things we want for ourselves and our nation. But to make that choice intelligently, we need to experience directly both the benefits and the costs of our choices. We especially need to prevent elected officials, drug companies, doctors, hospitals, advocacy groups, or anyone else from obscuring the benefits and costs to substitute their values for ours.

Three financial realities

There are some financial realities we have to take into consideration as we think about how to assign the costs of health care. The first reality we should take note of is that in almost any workable approach to broad health coverage, Americans who are better off economically have to subsidize the health care of those less well off. Other than adopting a third-world approach—a two-tier health care system in which those who can afford insurance buy it and those who can't default to a network of public clinics and hospitals, for example—it's hard to imagine how a system could work without such subsidies. Whenever a conservative throws the "You're redistributing wealth" charge at any new approach to health care financing, we should remind them we've already been quietly doing just that for almost a half century. We obviously do it in the Medicaid program, where the poor get medical care paid for by other citizens. But we've also been quietly and substantially doing it since the 1960s in the Medicare program as well. The payroll taxes paid into the Medicare trust fund quite obviously are greater for those with high incomes than those with low incomes. A substantial part of both Medicare Part B (the professional services part) and Part D (the pharmaceutical part) are paid from general tax revenues with their highly progressive structure. Many of the well-meaning folks who object to the "redistribution of wealth" in the Affordable Care Act either are or will be substantial beneficiaries of precisely that. The *extent* of the redistribution is open to debate. A legitimate ideological objection to the Affordable Care Act is the generous amount of it. But the *fact* of it is a long-established reality.

These subsidies for medical care are different from the way we treat other forms of social insurance. While Social Security has some redistribution of wealth built into its benefits, in large part the size of the Social Security check any of us will receive is directly related to what we put in over the years through our payroll taxes. Those who contribute more receive a larger benefit; those who contribute less, a smaller one. There's a similar relationship in private pension plans, or in the unemployment insurance that our employer pays on our behalf. Medical care is—and should be—different, at least for the basic care that we accept as a right of each American. If you walk down the corridor of a hospital today, the poor, the middle class, and the wealthy are all being treated to the same standard by the same people. We can and should debate the extent of the subsidy and the breadth of the items to which it should apply. But the first financial reality I want to put clearly in view is that, with health care, the wealthier have to subsidize those less wealthy to a greater extent than we see in other areas of our national life.

The second financial reality, and the most widely understood one, is that those of us who are well have to subsidize those who are sick. At any given time, 5% of the people are responsible for 50% of the costs. We've seen that health care has long ceased to fit a classic insurance model, but people do experience unexpected health care costs. There will always be accidents or unexpected diseases, and some protection against those costs is one of the things we want from our health care system. Furthermore, some people simply have higher health care costs throughout their lives, for reasons ranging from genetics or bad luck to their own personal choices. Even when those costs are a direct result of personal behaviors, as a matter of morality and practicality we still have to subsidize them. A thirty-five-year old with Type 2 diabetes brought on by his self-inflicted obesity is expensive to care for and he is unlikely to be able to pay the additional costs that result from his actions. Despite that, we're still going to treat him for his medical conditions. We're not going to let him die from heart disease or go blind if we can prevent it.

The third financial reality is less widely accepted but important in the overall financial picture of health care. We need to level the premiums paid by people of various ages. In simple terms, if you allow someone to purchase health insurance at a "fair value" while they're young, they're unlikely to be able to afford to purchase it at what would be a "fair value" later in life. As a practical matter, there has to be some subsidizing of older Americans by younger ones. The reason for this is how steeply health care costs rise with age. If you live to be eighty, in constant dollars you'll likely spend half your lifetime health care costs in your first sixty-five years, and the other half in the next fifteen. The contributions that any individual makes to health insurance premiums after the age of sixty-five (such as Medicare Part B premiums for physician services) are typically far less than the actual value of the insurance. This means that in a financially sustainable system everyone has to have established a substantial "savings account" before they retire. (Of course, as with Social Security, this is not literally a savings account but an intergenerational transfer—the young pay for today's elderly in exchange for the promise of being supported in turn when their time comes. But thinking about it as a savings account is a much clearer and perfectly valid view.)

It's easy to do a quick "back of the envelope" calculation to illustrate this. Insurance actuaries have established tables showing the relationship of the average cost of health care at various ages. As you might imagine, except for the very first year of life, the factor starts off quite low in the first couple of decades of one's lifetime (0.35 of the long-term average cost would be a typical ratio) and grows over time, reaching a nominal average (1.0) in the early forties. The growth then starts to speed up, with the age adjustment reaching around 3.0 at age sixty-five and 5.0 at age eighty.

Put another way, in the average person's eightieth year, his annual health care expenses would be expected to be on average about fifteen times what they were as a five-year-old, ten times what they were as a twenty-one-year-old, and five times what they were when he was in his early forties.

Now let me set a reasonable goal for myself: over my lifetime, I want to have paid for my own health care. During my working years (We'll say from age twenty-one to age sixty-five), I want to pay enough health insurance premiums to have repaid what was spent on me as a child, to take care of myself during my working years, and to have prepaid enough to pay for my health care in retirement. This is the absolute minimum of what my responsibility might reasonably be—I'm a working member of society and I'm planning to pay for at least my own health care. Of course, my real obligation on average is greater, as I might have a nonworking spouse, there may be times during my career when I'm not employed, and I have a social obligation to contribute to the health care of the poor.

The question is: in terms of what the "actuarially correct" premium would be to pay for my insurance in the middle of my life (I'm using my forty-second year), how much more do I have to put aside each year to meet this minimal standard of at least paying the lifetime costs for myself? You can work this out easily with a pencil and paper. The answer is that you have to put aside each year about 2.7 times the "*correct*" premium for your forty-second year. If that correct premium is $3,600 annually ($300 a month) then I need to actually pay $9,700 each year in order to repay what was provided me as a child and to build up an account, by the time I retire at sixty-five, of about $210,000. I'll then expect to draw that down to zero before I die, and will have left the world having taken "personal responsibility" for my own health care.

Obviously, that paper and pencil experiment is a great simplification, but it reflects the real costs of health care, and someone has to pay it. It could be me, someone on my behalf, someone with a higher income, or it could be borrowed from the Chinese government and paid back by my grandchildren. The point of the illustration is to show how difficult it is to just pay your own way, even if you start working hard at it when you're twenty-one. If you pay even less in those early years—an age adjusted premium—as the years go on it becomes more and more difficult even to pull your own weight.

A familiar face

I've described some financial realities that have to be taken into account when we start looking at how we pay for health care— the need to subsidize those with lower incomes, the need for the healthy to subsidize the ill, and the need to average costs across health status and age. Those principles may have a familiar ring to them. They should, as they're very similar to the workings of the most common health insurance of all—a traditional group health insurance plan. Whether in a corporation, a union trust fund, a nonprofit organization, or a unit of government, most Americans get their health insurance through these group plans, and the principles of subsidies and averaging that I've described are embodied in the way they operate.

A group health plan, in a sense, "subsidizes" lower income employees, in that the contribution of the employer is the same for every employee, and the contribution for lower income employees is a much larger fraction of their income than it is for a more highly compensated individual. The employer doesn't spread the value of this benefit across employees based on their worth to the organization (as indicated by their wages) but proportionally provides much more to lower income individuals.

A group health plan, while it may have waiting periods and exclusions, doesn't typically vary its premium to any great extent based on health status. Some are beginning to experiment with adjustments to premiums based on an employee's participation in desirable behavior (such as exercising) or undesirable behavior (such as smoking). The underlying structure of group health plans though is very much one man, one woman, one premium. Nor do group health plans vary their premiums by age. A twenty-five-year-old person who belongs to an employer-based plan pays the same premium as a sixty-four-year-old approaching retirement, even though their annual health care costs are very different.

In the pages ahead, keep this group health plan concept in mind. We'll make some changes and, especially, we'll incorporate much more powerful ways to control costs and improve quality, but the framework we'll start with is the group health plan. The employer (or union) group health plan is familiar, is well-liked, and has been around for a long time. Think of our starting point as a traditional group health plan on steroids. The "employer" becomes America, the "employee" becomes any American. We're going to design a group health plan for America.

The end of the company store

As we move forward, starting with the framework of a group health plan for America, we're leaving behind the familiar employer-sponsored health insurance. It's time to do this. As a society, we've long since abandoned the paternalism of the company store or company housing. There are doubtless a few examples still around at a mine site somewhere, or of necessity in the military, but most of us take our paychecks and decide where and how we want to spend them. When we need to buy something, we can go to Wal-Mart, or if we prefer, to Sears or Target or Neiman Marcus. Our employer provides a paycheck for the work we do, but the way in which we choose to spend it is our own.

Yet, for most Americans of working age, health care is still something deeply tied to the organization they work for. The employer decides, within wide parameters, the benefits to be offered and the suppliers (the insurance companies and the providers they contract with) who are allowed to offer it. This connection between health care and a person's employer has persisted over the years because, when it's stable, it works well. The problems arise when the employment relationship is broken for some reason. If a person leaves their employment voluntarily, or is laid off or fired, they and their family are disconnected from their health insurance as surely as they might have been from their family's company housing in the 1930s.

That reality has been brought home to many additional millions of Americans in our recent recession as they've been faced with the loss of their company-sponsored health insurance. Even with the help of Exchanges and generous subsidies in the Affordable Care Act, any change of insurance likely means a change in benefits, different financial arrangements, and, most important, the real possibility of a family member having to change doctors or other trusted providers. Similarly, family changes, whether through the breakup of a marriage or a death, is likewise often accompanied by a corresponding disconnection of health care relationships.

The provision of health insurance as a benefit of employment made more sense in a time when Americans expected to work for a single employer for very long periods of time, in many cases for a working lifetime. With every passing year, however, the American workforce becomes more and more mobile. My mother and several of her siblings worked for one employer for nearly all of their working lives. The experience of subsequent generations has been very different.

The concept of a group health plan for America breaks this connection once and for all. Employers, as we'll see, remain involved in the payment for health care just as they do with Social Security. But individuals will now have choice when it comes to health care. They'll decide where to purchase it completely independent of their relationship with any employer. It's no longer a "benefit" provided by someone else, it's something they own.

Can we trust government involvement in health care?

This is a big question and the answer isn't at all obvious. America has a great many individuals who have choices and are not dependent on the public sector for health insurance. Turning over much control of so personal a thing to Congress or HHS bureaucrats is a scary thing; I'm one of those Americans and it would be scary for me.

One thing is clear, however—when it comes to paying for health care, the role of government is inescapable. This role is already widely accepted: I've met few people, even very politically conservative ones, who think that Medicare should be scrapped. When I had to cut back our Medicaid program in Tennessee, opposition to those cuts came from Democrats and Republicans alike. The Affordable Care Act has further expanded that public role. Medicaid has been enlarged and the Act sets in place a broad array of federal subsidies for both individuals and businesses to help pay for health insurance. Government's role in generating revenue to pay for all this has expanded as well, with new taxes on both individuals and businesses and an assortment of charges to people and organizations that fail to participate. Long before the most recent reforms, a substantial role for government in paying for health care was firmly in place. Perhaps the pertinent question isn't *can* we trust it, but rather how to structure the role of government in a fashion that we *do* trust.

A real change has taken place in our level of trust even within my lifetime—the confidence that Americans place in their government today is quite different than it was for a couple of decades after World War II. A healthy skepticism is always appropriate (and very American) but paralysis isn't. Perhaps the reasons for this mistrust are the oft-cited ones: Vietnam, Watergate, Monica Lewinsky, Hurricane Katrina, cable news, and so on. But more likely the causes are deeper. Economic power, education, civil rights, the explosion of communication technologies and a host of other factors have made Americans more independent and more individualistic. In turn, we're less likely to see ourselves in terms of a relationship with any institution, whether it be a labor union, an employer, traditionally organized religion, or government itself.

There's an answer, though. With health care, there's a way that we could successfully address this trust issue and move forward. There are two distinct kinds of taxes in America. One kind we collect and use for all the varied purposes of general government. These are the income taxes, excise taxes, corporate taxes, and a great many more we use to fund the operation of our government: defense, diplomacy, Congress, research, regulation, justice, and thousands of other things. Let's call them the general taxes. The second kind of taxes are those designated for a specific purpose and generally set aside in a trust fund. Social Security and Medicare Part A (the part of Medicare that pays for hospital stays) are examples of these. These social insurance programs collect their revenue through a payroll tax and, at least from an accounting standpoint, segregate it in a trust fund that assures its use for a designated purpose. The federal fuel tax is another. It applies to motor fuels and is segregated in the Highway Trust Fund for use in the construction and maintenance of highways and bridges. Unemployment insurance is yet another. Let's call this second kind of taxes the trust fund taxes.

When we divide taxes into these two categories, it becomes clear that almost all of the distrust and antitax sentiment is directed at general taxes and the functions of government they support. This is where ideological differences play out, with disagreements about military spending, foreign aid, or services for the poor; this is where anger at $640 toilet seats or the antics of government officials is directed. The calls for tax cuts at the federal level are directed at these taxes. Conversely, very little of this distrust is directed at the trust fund taxes or at the things they pay for. It's only a small fringe element in our society who would want to cut Social Security or Medicare taxes and reduce the benefits they provide. There have been occasional calls in Congress to cut the fuel taxes that supply the federal Highway Trust Fund but they never go anywhere. In fact, in 1990 President George H. W. Bush signed legislation that increased the fuel tax and diverted half of the increase, not to building roads, but to general fund purposes to reduce the deficit. Within a decade this diversion was reversed by Congress, with the Taxpayer Relief Act of 1997, not by eliminating the tax being diverted but by restoring the full amount of the tax increase to the Highway Trust Fund for road and bridge construction. It would be hard to even imagine Congress cutting Social Security taxes and decreasing the benefits to match.

This confidence in trust fund taxes arises from two factors. First, with these, the connection between what any American pays and what they get is far more direct and understandable. Social Security taxes come back to you in a monthly check. Medicare taxes cover your hospital expenses if you should find yourself there after the age of sixty-five. Second, these trust fund taxes are seen as benefiting everyone. We'll all collect our Social Security and can be enrolled in Medicare when we reach the age at which we become eligible. We all drive on those roads and cross those bridges. We're not paying so that other people can get Social Security checks or drive on those roads, we're paying so that we can.

These trust funds are well-named: Americans do trust them. If there are good reasons to finance health care centrally, the use of a trust fund mechanism (which is very different from the way our present reform works) could be a politically workable approach. We'd collect the money we need for health care through broad and easily understood taxes, cleanly segregate the receipts in a trust fund, and pay that money out in as direct a fashion as possible to the same citizens who have paid it in. It's a simple and conservative approach we've already discovered and applied.

Vouchers

At this point, let's synthesize some more and set down a hypothesis about how a payment system might work. We'll take all the financial concepts we've been juggling—fairness, subsidies, economic tension, and more—and construct an approach. Then we'll check that approach against reality and see how it fares.

We'll begin with the concept that the proper role of government is to raise the money that it takes to run a comprehensive health care system, and then to back away and use the private sector—both nonprofit and for-profit—to deliver it. This is federal *financing* of health care but private *delivery*.

Here's the plan.

1. We'll collect the money we require for genuine universal health care through the tax system—as we'll see, through a combination of new payroll taxes and using the general tax system—and deposit it in a trust fund whose finances are completely segregated from those of general government. We'll require that the trust fund be actuarially sound at all times.

2. Each American will then have a voucher to purchase their health care from any system of care they choose. That voucher isn't tied to any specific employer or government program. My voucher is indistinguishable from that of an unemployed carpenter or a single mother who used to be a part of the Medicaid system. If you are a legal, breathing American you have one.

3. The health care that the voucher will buy will be the "standard" plan—a set of services that meet the reasonable medical care requirements of any individual, but stopping short of care that's discretionary: it's not the "gold" or "Cadillac" plan. Any individual or employer is free to add to these services at their own expense if they desire. Any state or local government is free to do the same. The systems of care

can offer these extras themselves, or they can be provided by third party organizations in much the same way Medicare "wraparound" insurance is provided today.

4. The idea of what constitutes "standard" coverage is rooted in our quality standards—in the Red Book—and is those things that the standards call for as appropriate treatment for the issue at hand. For these items, there's no coinsurance or deductibles; if it's care called for by the standards, it's paid for.

5. The value of each voucher is set annually and constitutes a cap on what we are willing to spend for that "standard" basket of health care services. The value is always tied to the actuarial soundness of the trust fund. If it's increased beyond what the trust fund can support, either as a political act or out of necessity, the supporting taxes have to be raised at the same time to keep the trust fund actuarially sound.

6. The way each person redeems their voucher is to use it to purchase membership in a specific licensed and regulated system of care. In order to obtain a license, a system of care would have to meet standards ensuring that they have a medical care system in place to deliver the package of services, would have to have the financial stability to guarantee their provision, and be able to meet standards of completeness and clarity in their descriptions of offerings to consumers. Each system of care will have its single quality score always prominently reported.

This approach of financing health care through the tax system, a trust fund, and issuing vouchers sweeps away a vast amount of complexity. First, and most important, it empowers individual citizens. Neither employers nor government controls one's health care choices, the individual does. My health coverage belongs to me and me alone; yours belongs to you and you alone; the same is true for every one of our three hundred million plus citizens. Our coverage and relationship with our doctors is undisturbed through the expected and unexpected twists and turns of life. We can change employers, we can become unemployed and reemployed, we can get married and separated and divorced, or our spouses can change jobs, but through all this our health care arrangements remain under our complete control. Each American will have great personal choice in what system of care they trust and prefer—much more than now. If they do make a change, it's their decision and not an accident of circumstance. How much we pay into the trust fund adjusts automatically to our circumstances, without the need for intrusive questions or trips to any human services office.

This approach also sweeps away a broad array of issues that we've piled solution upon complicated solution trying to solve. There is no longer a need for Americans to go through an elaborate and often demeaning process of applying to a bureaucracy for assistance based on income or any other status. Nor is there a need for the vast bureaucracy itself. The whole process of subsidizing care is naturally and simply self-adjusting: those with lower income will automatically pay less and those with higher will automatically pay more. The entire Medicaid program and its vast apparatus simply disappears. While we'd need an extended transition time, the Medicare system is transformed and integrated with the rest of health care. The issue of enforcement of mandates or of discovering the inevitable cheating in the subsidized system for payment goes away as well. The reporting and payment of income and payroll taxes is a simple and well-established part of the employment process and the monitoring apparatus is already in place. There are no more uninsured Americans, and so the whole system of supplemental payments to providers to compensate them for unpaid care—diminished but far from eliminated by the Affordable Care Act—is no longer needed.

There's no complex system of limiting out-of-pocket payments to a certain portion of income: it's no longer needed.

How much do we need?

So far, we've talked about a different approach to gathering and distributing the money that it takes to pay for health care in conceptual terms. As the next step, we'll look at what this means in more specific terms. In this discussion, we'll use figures for the year 2007; that's the last year for which comprehensive actual data is available and the last "normal" year before the distortions of the recession began to be felt. We'll update our numbers at the end to a more useful point in time, to reflect both the Patient Protection and Affordable Care Act and the considerable inflation that will have occurred during the intervening years.

First, we'll see how much money in total is needed. We'll start with the amount of money that would be needed to just exactly match what we're spending now and add those who are in 2007 uninsured, with no allowances for savings that might be accomplished. Second, we'll consider what changes would be needed to our tax system to assemble it.

The federal Department of Health and Human Services maintains extensive data on national health expenditures, and we'll use their data as our starting point. In 2007, we spent $2.241 trillion for health care in the United States. Included in that total are a number of expenditures that would not be included in a national health care plan. For example, we should obviously keep our public health and medical research expenditures separate and plan to continue them as before. I've also excluded nursing home expenditures in the belief that they need to be dealt with in another fashion. The approach I'm describing could be extended to include them if desired. There are a number of categories of health expenditures where we would not expect to cover all of the services accounted for in a national plan: the

Department of Defense provides medical care for personnel overseas, the Department of Veterans Affairs offers specialized services for veterans in addition to general medical care, and a considerable amount of dental care and most cosmetic surgery fall outside of the scope of the services we would want to cover.

Once we've established a baseline of how much we're spending now (in 2007 for this example) on services that would be candidates for inclusion in our comprehensive plan, we need then to add to that the new costs we'd expect as we make available coverage to those who are uninsured. This is a difficult number to determine. There are direct government appropriations to some providers to pay them for otherwise uncompensated care, primarily through the Medicaid system. But there's also considerable cost shifting to other parties through prices they are charged that are higher than they might be otherwise. Most difficult of all is estimating what health services are not being provided today but will be when the patient has the ability to pay for them.

A careful and neutral study of what additional costs would be needed to cover the uninsured was done by the Kaiser Commission on Medicaid and the Uninsured. The authors took into account the factors I've described and also included estimates of the actual health status of the uninsured and their demographics. That study concluded that the incremental cost in 2008 would be about $123 billion. (That number passes a reasonableness check: if you inflate it suitably and see what it totals to in the 2014–2019 years that were priced by the CBO for the recent health reform, the Kaiser estimate would be about $1.2 trillion over that period. Health reform addresses about two-thirds of the total number of uninsured, and two-thirds of $1.2 trillion is $800 billion, which roughly corresponds to the costs that CBO determined for that portion of reform.)

If we deflate the Kaiser number by a year to correspond it to our 2007 base year, we'd have to add about $116 billion to bring it up to the level where we would be able to cover everyone. I've arbitrarily assigned that cost to the private and government sectors in the same proportion as they share existing costs. When all this is done, what results is that we need about $2.0 trillion to pay for health care, and the breakdown is that $1.2 trillion is coming from the private sector, $600 billion from the federal government (including Medicare taxes and premiums), and $200 billion from state and local governments. On a per capita basis, it's $6,650 for each individual in the United States. All of this is summarized in Table 5.

Table 5
National health expenditures (2007) for inclusion in national care
$ billions

		Private	Federal	State/Local	Total
Total		1,206	754	281	2,241
Less:	Public Health		(10)	(54)	(64)
	Research	(4)	(33)	(5)	(42)
	Nursing Home	(50)	(57)	(25)	(132)
	Industrial In-Plant	(8)			(8)
	Dept of Defense		(38)		(38)
	Philanthropy				0
	Veterans Admin at 50%		(41)		(41)
	Cosmetic Surgery	(8)			(8)
	Dental at 50%	(21)			(21)
	TOTALS	1,115	575	197	1,887
Now add in cost of uninsured and spread in same proportion		69	35	12	116
	GRAND TOTAL	1,184	610	209	2,003
	Population of the U.S. (millions)	301.3			
	Per Capita Contribution	3,928	2,026	694	6,648

Source: http://www.cms.gov; National Health Expenditure Data; file NHE_2007_V8.csv

How do we assemble $2.0 trillion?

First, let's set one of the possibilities aside. One approach would be to echo the payroll tax that Social Security and Medicare Part A depend on. Total wage and salary income in 2007 was about $6.1 trillion, so if a tax were levied on all such income (without the wage limitations of Social Security taxes) it would need to be 33% of wage and salary income. If we were to place limitations on the incomes to which this applies, the percentage goes even higher. This doesn't work: no one is likely to want to impose a 33% tax on the wages of an individual making a median income of $32,000 annually (even though it's *still* a bargain; if you have even a single dependent, your actual share of health care costs is more than the $10,500 that your 33% payroll tax would produce). As a practical matter, we have to make how we pay for health care far more progressive, and the way to do that is to bring into play more progressive sources of taxation. (This example, however, shows just how deep the water we've gotten into is when it comes to health care expenses in America.)

Bringing other parts of our tax system into play has to depend substantially on the personal income tax, which amounts to about 70% of all federal revenues outside of the existing payroll taxes. This is a highly progressive tax, with 97% of all personal income taxes paid by the top half of taxpayers (those earning above or about $50,000) and 60% of all tax paid by the top five percent (those earning above about $165,000). Modifying the personal income tax by itself won't solve the problem either, as the total amount paid in personal income tax in 2007 was $1.2 trillion, far less than the cost of health care.

The other possible sources of revenue based on the existing system are the corporate income tax (about 19% of total federal non-payroll taxes) and excise taxes (a little under 5%). Either of these could be a contributor to the total, but neither are large enough to carry a substantial part of the load. Of course, if the United States were to substantially modify its tax system—a flat tax, or some form of consumption tax such as a value-added tax—the analysis would change. I'm assuming for this discussion that we're working with the kinds of taxes that are in general use today.

The concept that I want to offer is straightforward, and has probably occurred to you by now. We've broken down the components of health expenditures into three parts: state government, federal, and private. The big change we'll make is to replace the private component, which includes all the various premiums paid by individuals and employers for health insurance, with a straightforward addition to existing payroll taxes. In our base 2007 year, total salaries and wages paid were $6.141 trillion, and so in its simplest terms—a starting place—this would require an additional 19.3% Federal Insurance Contribution Act tax (FICA) contribution, or about $7,900 for an American with an average $41,000 wage. If that cost were split between an employer and employee in a typical ratio of three-quarters to the employer and one-quarter to the employee, that would mean an annual cost to the employee of a little under $2,000, or about $165 per month. (Of course, to be strictly fair, the employer cost is also paid by the employee as well, in that those costs might well displace additional wages or other benefits that the employer might have been able otherwise to provide.)

Let me instantly acknowledge that the mere idea of a payroll tax that collects an additional 19% of salary and wages will cause a great many people to begin hyperventilating. It shouldn't, though. This is not a new expenditure, it just replaces the contributions to conventional health insurance that are being made today by a great many employers and employees. In the form I've just described it, middle income citizens will actually experience a *decrease* in what they're paying right now for health care. If our average (in 2007) $41,000 employee has a family health insurance plan, it's total cost might be about $11,000 annually, and the employees share might typically be 25% of that, or $230 per month. The $165 a month that this approach represents is substantially less. Likewise, that average worker's employer is now paying $687 per month as their share and that would go down to about $500.

While that might seem counterintuitive, there are two things going on to make it possible. First, the levy of the payroll taxes is much broader in that it includes people and businesses who don't now pay them (and many who will not under the Patient Protection and Affordable Care Act). Many of these are small businesses and many of them will viscerally dislike the idea of such a payroll tax and claim that it will bankrupt them. I truly love small businesses—I've worked in them, my wife operated one for years, my son works for a small business, and my father has owned and worked at one for most of his working life (and still does at age ninety-two). But they need to be reasonable. If everyone is paying the same, it's no competitive disadvantage any more than Social Security is. Economists will predict some job losses (as they do with raising the minimum wage) but there will also be enormous job creation and many other opportunities as a result of these changes to the health care system. Most of all, there's simple fairness. We don't give small businesses and their employees any special consideration on their income taxes. Everybody who earns the same income pays the same. We charge everyone the same Social Security and Medicare taxes: a percentage of their income. I understand the impulse for a small business to want special consideration—everyone wants that. But the structure of taxes needs to be on a firmer foundation than the number of employees a particular business employs.

Second, this payment system is much more progressive than the insurance system it replaces. An employee who has a $250,000 income today pays the same amount for health insurance as one with a $50,000 income, but under an uncapped payroll tax system would pay considerably more—in the nominal situation, five times more. The wages to which the tax applies could be capped at some amount just as we cap the wage base for Social Security taxes. It's particularly appropriate in the case of health care, as the higher income employee will also be paying substantial income taxes that contribute to paying for health care as well.

Within this basic concept there are many ways to fine-tune the share of health care payments that would be borne by people at various levels of income. The payroll tax doesn't have to be a flat tax like Medicare or Social Security; it could be at one rate for income up to a certain level, and another above that level. We can change the proportion of total expenses collected through a payroll tax, rather than changing the federal income tax system, to make the payment for health care more or less progressive and to capture more or less of the income that doesn't flow through a payroll check, such as various kinds of investment income. We can add modest copayments for some kinds of services to off-load a portion of the private contribution from the payroll tax system.

We'll explore in the next chapter how this might look in specific terms as a part of our overall health care plan. But if we can summon the political will to make a change of this sort, it transforms so much about our health care system. We would genuinely empower our citizens, disengaging health coverage from being something provided by an employer, a government program, or a combination of both; it becomes a right possessed by each individual. What any individual contributes toward payment for their health care depends on their income only, and is adjusted up or down, or eliminated, in the easiest and most natural way possible. No one has to fill out forms and apply for anything, no outsider need know their income, and there are no opportunities to lie or to forget to keep the government informed of every change in income or other status. Providers of medical care would be blind to the finances of their patients and would be paid the same for their services to a poor person as for the same services to a doctor or a lawyer.

This is our sixth and final stepping-stone—a complete redesign of the payment for health care. This final stone is a longer step—abandoning the ponderous collection of various payment systems we've accumulated and replacing them with something simple and fair.

Final thoughts

As I come to the end of this chapter, I feel the need to explain just a little further the approach I'm advocating. My political philosophy and approach to governing has been by any standard a fiscally conservative one. The property tax rate was lower in Nashville at the end of my term as mayor than it was at the beginning; as governor I've guided the state through two very difficult fiscal times not with new or increased taxes but with deep cuts in our spending. Through those times, we've kept our finances strong—our borrowings are among the lowest per capita in the nation and are not used to support operating expenses. We have recently achieved a AAA bond rating. Despite the severe recession, we still have strong cash reserves and an actuarially sound pension fund. When we needed to deal with ballooning costs in our Medicaid system, we dealt with the issue and made cuts, making enemies for me within my own political party who persist to this day. Yet it would be easy to get the impression that I close this chapter having just proposed an enormous tax increase.

But I haven't. With the exception of the money to expand coverage to the uninsured that I've added (and which is already largely included now in our recent reform) we've not added one dollar to the costs of health care. What we've done is just to take all the money that is being spent right now—through an impenetrable thicket of complex and inconsistent ways—and set it down in front of us where we can see it, evaluate it, and take control of it.

The concept of fiscal conservatism has been cheapened these past years; it's come to be synonymous with just being against anything that can be called a tax. It's a bigger and more constructive concept than that. Those of us in politics should be frugal and judicious in the way we spend the public's money, but we should also be honest about what we're doing and we should above all protect the independence and wealth of our nation. That's the real fiscal conservatism.

12

Putting It All Together

. . . in which we explore how we might move forward with our concepts in the world of practical politics. We first establish the quality assurance system, which will be valuable however we proceed in the future. Next, we establish the framework for systems of care and begin their development. Finally, we prepare ourselves for the inevitable crisis—the black swan event—which will provide the political energy to permanently alter the financing and organization of health care.

We've been working our way to a better system of health care as if we were crossing a stream; stepping carefully on one solid rock at a time. First stepping-stone: establish a framework for fairness and dignity. Second: understand just *why* health care is so expensive. Third: find a better way to manage very large and loosely connected organizations—hypercomplexity. Fourth: elevate quality of care—conforming to evidence-based standards—to the central role. Fifth: use integrated systems of care as our fundamental unit of organization. Sixth and final: rationalize the payment—a broad payroll and income tax, a trust fund, and vouchers. We've advanced across each of these stepping-stones, and we're now at a place where we can step onto the far bank.

There's always the possibility that there could be a circumstance that would let us assemble all of this together in one piece and move forward. I think it just possible that President Obama might have been able to accomplish this with some variant of what I've laid out had he made a different set of choices at the outset. There's always the chance of the right confluence of a leader and a time that would again make it possible. But that's a long shot, depending on too many tumblers clicking into place at just the right time. Moreover, the reform we've just passed has released much of the energy around changing the health system, and a public weary of it is now turning to other things. That's not all bad, though.

We've just finished a process of designing a solution for a complicated problem by breaking it up into sequential pieces—our stepping-stones—and that could be a strong way to implement it as well. With any complex effort, it's always a good thing to get something simple together, get it into operation in the real world, and then use the feedback from that to design the next iteration. We've all become familiar with software terms these past years—in those terms I'd say: get version 1.0 out the door, into the hands of your customers, and then learn from that to design version 2.0. Working diligently to design version 4.0 perfectly, without that iterative process, is likely to ensure that the product never sees the light of day, and if it does, that it misses the mark by a long way.

When Tim Berners-Lee sat down and invented the World Wide Web, he didn't try to imagine and provide for Amazon, let alone Google. Perhaps late at night alone with his desk lamp he permitted himself a daydream or two about where his child might go, but he didn't let that divert him or slow him down. He wrote down a simple set of protocols—a framework—that could be expanded, got it all working, and let the world have at it. Over time, others used the simple framework he provided to build on his ideas in ways he never imagined and never could have

imagined: Internet shopping, search engines, news, online bank-
ing, Facebook, Wikipedia, YouTube, eBay, and millions of others.
The American health care system is, of course, very different: it
doesn't exist in one man's mind, it's a sixth of the biggest economy
in the world. There are deeply entrenched economic interests, and
we're far enough down the wrong road that it will require taking
some things back, always extremely difficult. Launching changes
to health care is vastly more difficult than Professor Berners-Lee
setting up the first Web server on a little desktop computer. But
the underlying principles can guide us.

We need a simple framework, and we have one: citizens armed
with health care vouchers, and systems of care to receive them,
ever balancing the tension between the money they have, the audited quality of the care they provide, and the satisfaction of their
customers. Everything else—where the vouchers come from, how
big they are, exactly how we audit the care, just how the systems
of care work and are organized—will evolve over time, doubtless
in ways none of us even imagine today. But as long as we keep the
underlying framework intact, we'll have control over our costs and
our citizens will get high quality health care.

The question is: how do we get that framework launched into
the world; how do we get version 1.0 born? Especially, how do
we do so in a way that can actually be accomplished in the real
world of politics, and how can the integrity of that framework be
sustained across more than one president, or Congress, or control
by any particular political party? I propose we tackle this practical
problem in three steps.

Step 1: the quality metric

The first step seems obvious and relatively easy. Right now,
without even any further commitment to the framework we've described, the system for establishing standards and auditing them
should be set up. Whatever directions health care takes over the

years, it's hard to imagine one in which a robust system of quality standards and the measurement of real world care against them would not be a priceless asset. The quality auditing process is one of the essential gears in the system. It'll take time for us to build it and work out the problems. We want this embedded as a permanent part of our new system of health care, and the way to make that happen is to make it routine.

We're in a good position to start this. The belief in "evidence-based medicine" is strong and the importance of its role in the future of health care is already reflected in the Affordable Care Act. What's still lacking is a process to give it real substance. Establishing standards—the Red Book—is a natural extension of things already underway today and one that would be seen as sensible by many people. There will, of course, be opposition to the idea from many practitioners, but some of those arguments are inevitable as we move ahead. No one likes change, especially change that puts a spotlight on where there had been none before. However, there's no better place to stand politically when having that argument than to simply insist the profession itself develop and write down clear and quantifiable quality standards for the practice of medicine.

The American Medical Standards Panel—the Red Book authors— would be a good first step for the changes we'll want to make over the years. The concept is understandable to everyone. It starts the practice of medicine down the path of establishing independent science as the gold standard and not just the inconsistencies of "professional judgment." The process of establishing standards will quickly highlight areas where research (and discussion) is needed, and that in turn can be gotten underway. The Red Book is a warm-up: an easy way for everyone to start familiarizing themselves with a new approach to health care. It lets everyone start moving their muscles in a new way. It's inexpensive and almost risk-free, but capable of launching profound changes in how medicine is practiced. It's also a warm-up for Congress: to give them some practice and work through the issues of setting up components of our new system with the genuine independence they need to be successful.

The American Medical Standards Panel can also be the basis for tackling another problem in medical care—tort reform. If medical practitioners were afforded a "safe harbor" when care that conforms to the standards is competently provided, a lot of problems could be solved. It moves the discussion of an appropriate standard of care from the flawed world of dueling "experts" arguing complex and indeterminate issues in front of a jury, to a far calmer and more appropriate one. Such an approach still protects the right of a patient to seek redress in court for genuine wrongs. If a doctor acts in a way that disregards established medical standards or incompetently performs the care set out there, he is still subject to the actions of an injured party. It gives good doctors real protection and is a far more delicately tuned instrument than arbitrary caps on damages.

As we discussed earlier, in order to give the panel the imprimatur it needs, we'll set it up as a government chartered but independent agency. Appointing such a body is always difficult, but an approach in which a rotating group of academic medical centers made dual appointments, one from within and one external to themselves and to academia, would be a good starting place. We could likewise add appointments from a rotating group of the major professional societies, and a small number as presidential appointments from the nation as a whole. If I were asked to be specific, I might recommend a seventeen-member committee. Ten of the members would be appointed by five academic medical centers taken randomly from a list of twenty selected by a vote of the nation's medical schools. Each academic institution would select one member from their own organization and one from outside of academia. Five of the members would likewise be chosen from a rotating group of the major professional societies, and two would be presidential appointments.

There are obviously many variations on just how such a panel might be structured. There are two elements that are essential, however. First, the panel needs to be expert and disinterested. This is not the place to award every interest group—economic or professional—its own position. And second, its financing will be modest, but needs to be outside of the appropriations process and thereby gain some insulation from political pressure.

With a standards committee underway, we would then move on to setting up the National Independent Quality Audit. Here, the National Committee for Quality Assurance (NCQA) would be a good starting point and central dispatch. As we discussed in Chapter 9, the process will be to sample medical records from providers across the nation, to ensure that the sample is appropriate for the data that is being looked at, and then to abstract them and make them anonymous.

You'll remember that the Quality Audits themselves would be performed by independent auditing organizations around the country. We could start with a few such organizations—say five—and then expand as we work out the problems and approaches we are going to use. NCQA would be responsible for setting these up through a competitive process and monitoring the results. These organizations receive the selected records on a random basis, process them against the Red Book standards, and report the results back to NCQA. We haven't yet set up formal systems of care, so we won't be ready yet to report the single scores that we're seeking later on. But there is no reason why the predecessors of our systems of care—insurance companies, hospitals, and other provider organizations—shouldn't have access to the data privately. They can start identifying where their problems are likely to be, gain experience with the system, and provide valuable feedback to the entire effort. These Quality Audits will quickly produce a rich lode of information that can be used by individuals, insurers, providers, and employers in many ways.

The funding for this effort is a simple fee on the fiscal intermediaries, including those handling Medicare and Medicaid. In exploring the idea earlier, we looked at a 0.25% fee on all medical transactions and saw that it produced enough funding to operate a comprehensive program without adding substantially to the cost of care. In fact, this level of quality monitoring would simply, by its presence, likely create savings many times greater than its cost. We'll want, for simplicity and efficiency, to limit our fee to fiscal intermediaries and so will miss some of the cost of the transactions for now—such as co-pays, deductibles, and various private pay transactions. Even with that, it will take time to set up and put in operation this quality system, and a fee at the intermediary level will grow as the system evolves to a higher reliance of systems of care and ultimately to a voucher system in which nearly all the revenue is captured.

Any time that new fees are proposed, there's guaranteed to be consternation. But in this particular case the intermediaries—insurance companies, HMOs, and so on—would find this information extremely desirable to have, unobtainable in any other practical way and therefore likely to be supportive. Even more important, the employers who are paying for much of the care would find quality information of this depth very valuable. They could use it in managing their insurance programs, selecting vendors for administrative and management services, and devising new payment mechanisms. As insurers and employers are the two directly affected private parties, a small percentage fee to finance a comprehensive quality audit effort could be relatively easy to put in place. We'll start out at 0.125% and set it up to grow to a full 0.25% over a five-year period.

Step 2: systems of care

The next step, after we have the standards and auditing component underway, would be for Congress to formally establish a legislative framework for systems of care. Like our quality assurance system, these, too, will take time to set up and we'll benefit from some experience with them before we trust them with our entire health care system.

There are several things to be accomplished.

First, we'll set up the areas in which the systems of care will operate. I'll call them Integrated Health Service Areas (IHSAs). We want them to reflect the underlying reality of population distributions and travel habits and to be large enough to support three or four competing systems of care. They should also be designed to integrate the demographics of a region; we want each system to have a mix of urban and rural patients, and to have poor, middle-class, and wealthy patients. Nothing will drive health care quality to poor and underserved parts of our nation as quickly as having their quality measurements lumped together with those of desirable and wealthy suburbs.

The systems of care will obviously cut across state lines. The U.S. Office of Management and Budget has defined 942 "core based statistical areas," and combining these rationally to produce 250 or 300 cores for our IHSAs would be a good start We'd then take the resulting boundaries and expand them until they touched each other and covered the entire United States. There would be some outliers to be dealt with due to size or geography: Alaska, for example.

The legislation would then set up the standards for what constitutes a system of care—financial viability, the scope and completeness of the delivery system, and so on. The systems would be licensed at the state level and states would be responsible for their regulation.

The provision of medical care today is governed by a state-by-state hodgepodge of laws, regulation, and boards that, if left intact, would inhibit the innovations by systems of care we need. A fundamental principle of the approach I'm proposing is to measure systems of care by their results—their quality scores—and not their means. In almost every state, there are laws and regulations that have been imposed over the years to protect or grant economic advantage for some group of providers. Some states, for example, have "any willing provider" laws. These laws guarantee that if an insurance company negotiated a lower cost contract with a pharmacy chain, they would also have to contract with any other pharmacy willing to meet the lower price. This of course removes most of the point of negotiating prices, doubtless the intent of those proposing the law in the first place. Systems of care can lower prices for drugs if they can simply use normal negotiating techniques for their purchase.

Or, as another example, if a system of care were to work with a physician group to arrange for some kinds of prescriptions to be dispensed in the physician's office, they should be free to do so without running afoul of laws forbiding it (wouldn't it be convenient to just have the pediatrician's nurse give you that antibiotic prescription for your child?). This clearing out of the accumulated brush in the legal environment of medical care will be contentious, but is essential and best handled right at the outset.

What Congress will need to accomplish is to pass legislation that sets up systems of care and provides standards for licensure that help ensure the safety of their patients but leave them the maximum possible discretion in how they meet those standards. They'll need to sweep aside the state laws that have encrusted medical care with protectionism and unnecessary regulation and provide the fluid environment that will encourage innovation and cost saving.

At this point, Congress will have set up the legal framework but there are as yet no patients. As the last step of this second phase, Congress should also alter the Medicaid program so that systems of care can freely be used to provide those services. It's critical to change the underlying legislation and not depend on the granting of "waivers" by the Medicaid bureaucracy. Everyone needs to be able to play by the same rules and to move confidently without the limitations, arbitrariness, and limited time horizons that constrain innovation in Medicaid today. States struggling with these costs may well be the first to turn to systems of care. They can be the early adopters who spur the actual creation of the first systems of care, build up valuable experience with millions of patients, and get them ready for the major role we've prepared for them.

Step 3: end game

Now, most probably, we wait a bit.

One possibility is that the systems of care will prove themselves able to provide better care at lower costs, and gradually more and more people will move into them. Medicaid will use them, and perhaps Medicare or the subsidized insurance plans brokered by the exchanges will provide incentives to use them. Almost certainly there will be employers who will move their employees to them. Such gradual adoption would be a disappointment: the existing insurance-based system will continue to exist alongside and will provide a convenient ceiling for pricing and a status quo alternative for providers. Health maintenance organizations suffered that fate: existing insurance plan rates provided a lazy price umbrella and they never became hungry enough (or had the flexibility we're giving our systems of care) to truly change the way medical care was delivered.

The second alternative is to go ahead and take the last step: change the entire financing mechanism to a trust fund and vouchers, and deliver all essential medical care through systems of care. Perhaps there will be the political will simply to go ahead and do this. It has elements that could appeal to a range of ideologies: for the left, true universal coverage and far greater dignity for the poor; for the right, believable cost control and a private sector and market-based solution; for everyone, far more ownership and control over their health care.

However, it's one of life's rules that we most often make the big changes only when there's a crisis. We all know people who have made very large changes in their lifestyle, and we've also likely observed that it happens when something jolts or scares them into doing it—a heart attack, a stroke, a DUI conviction, a family intervention. A crisis might be what jolts us into finishing the transition. He wasn't the first to observe it, but Rahm Emanuel said it well: "You never let a serious crisis go to waste. And what I mean by that is it's an opportunity to do things you think you could not do before."

I've already noted that we are very far out on the financial limb in our country and aren't worried nearly enough about it. All the projections we see, with whatever level of optimism or pessimism they contain, are nice smooth curves. They assume a smooth and predictable development in the years ahead. We develop projections that go out ten and twenty years with a subversive precision, forgetting that being able to use Excel doesn't make us smart. We calculate our ratio of debt to our gross national product and I guess we assume that at some point, Congress will get up out of the chair and do something about it (even though that "something" is rapidly getting draconian indeed). More than likely, that's not the way it'll play out.

Nassim Taleb has made famous the logician's old idea of the "black swan"—the importance of what we falsely believe to be impossible or highly improbable events. His idea is that our narrative minds place far too much importance on continuity and on the past as a guide to the future when in fact the big events—the "game changers"—are unpredictable and show up completely unexpectedly. He offers the example (among others) of September 11—completely unexpected, shocking, and world-changing. As he observes, "History does not crawl, it jumps." He wrote about his ideas before the latest black swan event, but all of us who recently lived through all those trillions of dollars of bulletproof AAA-rated bonds becoming worthless (and the resulting near-collapse of the world financial system) find this view of the way things were believable.

This last step in fixing our health care system will probably occur in response to a new black swan event. We'll need a serious crisis, when there are suddenly compelling reasons to do tough things to fix our finances and the political will to take the steps necessary. It could be an upheaval in China (there have already been a couple in my adult lifetime), the failure of some part of the European Union financial system (or for that matter, California's), or in the spirit of black swan events, something else totally unexpected. It seems highly probable, though, that at some not too distant time we'll be faced with a crisis that will force us to fix our country's finances. I believe our citizens will understand, perhaps before their elected officials, that it can't be done without fixing our entitlements.

When it happens, we need to have thought through our response and have a framework to guide us. When it comes to health care, our nation has too many very smart people and the stakes are far too high to leave this to Congress—running around, inventing on the fly and under pressure to pass "a budget reform bill," whatever that means. We'll need to have thought this through ahead of time.

The final pieces

If we've taken the first two steps—setting up the quality audits and the systems of care—then the third and final step is straight-forward: Congress legislatively creates the trust fund, defines the taxes that support it, and sets the annual amount of the vouchers. There are many variations on how this might be structured, but to illustrate, let me select one as a starting point.

- We'll start in 2016 and give ourselves fifteen years—through 2030—to make the full transition. Our goal will be that health care represent no more than 14% of the U.S.

economy at the end of this transition and the cost of health care after that will grow at no more than the rate of the economy itself. If we achieve this goal, in 2030 our annual national health care costs will be about $4 trillion less than the track we're now on and over the fifteen year transition period, we'll spend about $25 trillion less on health care than we're now planning. This is real change.

- We'll design a payment system for our trust fund so that when we come to the year 2030, it will pay for 100% of the standard care Americans are guaranteed and there will be no unfunded future liabilities. During the interim, in order to make the transition feasible, we'll borrow to make up the difference between the initial revenues our trust fund will receive and the actual costs. These borrowings will total about $6 to $7 trillion over the fifteen year period and will represent about 20% of the projected 2030 GDP. That's our working capital to make the changes we need.

- We'll set the initial voucher rates at 100% of current costs for the standard services and then constrain the total amount of the vouchers to grow at a rate equal to one-half the rate of growth of the economy for the fifteen year period. That strategy will get us slightly under the 14% of GDP target for overall health care costs. Remember that we've eliminated some health care costs from the trust fund process—research, for example—and so the amount being financed in this way is somewhat less, about 89% of the total.

- For those areas of the country where health care expenses are in excess of the national average, the voucher amount increases will be held at zero until they reach the average. For those where expenses are lower, we'll be more generous with the annual increases so that they grow by 2030 to the average.

- We'll provide the trust fund with revenues through a payroll tax of 10% of the first $30,000 and 20% thereafter, up to a maximum of $500,000 of wage or salary income. The existing Medicare taxes will be included in those amounts, so it represents new contributions of about 7% and 17% respectively. We'll allocate those taxes 75% to the employer and 25% to the employee, which reflects a typical split in a group health plan today.

- We'll incorporate the federal contribution as an income tax surcharge of 20%. If these funds can be provided for in other ways through the federal system without borrowing, that's fine as well.

- We'll continue a state contribution of the present 12.5% of the total, adjusted state by state according to the FMAP formula (to take into account a state's personal income compared with the rest of the country).

Let's pause a moment here, as almost anyone reading the structure that I've just laid out for paying for health care will be taken aback. A *twenty percent* payroll tax? And a *twenty percent* surcharge on income taxes? But, as we saw in the last chapter, for most middle income Americans who have employer-sponsored health insurance today—which is most middle-income Americans—this actually represents a *decrease* in what they and their employers would already be paying. At the time of our assumed start date of 2016, a typical family health insurance plan will be in the range of $15-16,000 annually. For a person making $60,000 annually with such a typical insurance plan, the $12,000 annually that the payroll tax represents plus the roughly $1,000 annually that the income tax surcharge would cost them is considerably less than that. Fifteen years later, in 2030, it's dramatically less than they'd be paying. Of course, for those with much higher incomes, this represents a genuine and substantial increase. The approach I've postulated has to be quite progressive in order to keep the costs for lower income workers under control.

In fact, to keep the cost as low as I've sketched the trust fund has to be combined with some very aggressive—draconian—cost management. This level of cost management would, if possible at all, only be so with sensible nationwide limitations on the on the amount of money available and very strong financial incentives in play. As a point of reference, if we just let health care costs continue to rise at the rates now projected, it would take a payroll tax above 30% and a 50% income tax surcharge to balance the books in 2030. And even more in 2040.

If you don't like the numbers I've sketched, that's fine. If 14% of GDP is too low in your estimation, pick another percentage. If 20% of payroll is too high and you want more of the costs borne by the rich, pick a lower payroll tax number and increase the income tax surcharge. The only rule is that you have to balance the books. If we're determined, in the end, to pay our way—as we're going to have to do—it's going to take disciplined, strong, and difficult action on both the payment and the cost control side of the health care equation.

Years ago, when I had my first chance as a young business executive to turn around a failing business, my boss gave me some advice. It wasn't original—it's been repeated in a million different ways over the years—but no less sage for that. The way he told it to me was, "If you do what you always did, you'll get what you always got." The finances of our health care system are very much in a turnaround situation. I don't know where my old boss is these days, but Washington could profit from his advice.

Vouchers

Once the trust fund and its revenue base is designed, we can move on to the design of the vouchers themselves. We'd want the amount of the vouchers to vary in three ways. They need to be adjusted by age and sex as both have a significant impact on health care costs; if we don't adjust them we invite the systems of care to game us with selective marketing.

We would also need to vary the vouchers by a regional cost-of-living index to reflect the different costs of doing business across the nation. This is specifically *not* a health care cost index adjustment, as we're going to eliminate, not encourage, the regional differences that exist in health care costs. But it's more expensive in general to operate an organization in Boston than in Nashville and that ought to be recognized. As a matter of fairness, a higher voucher value in Boston is partially compensated for by higher salaries there as well, and therefore higher contributions on average to the health care trust fund.

In the short term, we'll plan to add some additional modifications to the various voucher amounts, and then remove those differences over a period of time. We've already noted that there are large and unjustified regional differences in the cost of medical care. It would be excessively disruptive to both providers and patients to instantly eliminate those and the plan I set out eliminates them over time. In the initial stages, it would also make sense to vary the voucher amounts in a few broad ways to reflect the health status of incoming patients. There are several reasons for this. We'll want to encourage large integrated hospital systems to become systems of care, but they will also have a large number of sick patients who are familiar with them, seeing physicians associated with them and likely to join their system of care. There will also be a small number of patients with very high and long-term health costs—patients with spinal or head injuries, for example—and it would make sense to recognize those at the outset as well.

This initial setting of voucher rates based on health status should be done very conservatively, however. There is always the danger of an epidemic of "upcoding" where lots of patients are suddenly found to be much sicker than they had previously been thought to be. And while we accept today that a person with diabetes costs the health care system more because of that disease, we want the system of care to be under considerable economic pressure to manage the disease more efficiently, and not just recognize and institutionalize those costs in the payment system.

These and doubtless other adjustments will be needed to allow a smooth transition, but we want to ensure that we are always moving toward a simple system. Before too many years go by, we want everyone treated the same; their vouchers varying by age, sex, and where they are located. Every system of care will have patients everywhere on the axis from those who rarely use the medical care system to the very sick. It's their job to provide excellent, appropriate care to all of them and to do so within the budgets set by the vouchers.

The far shore

Here's the health care system we have now envisioned:

- Every American—throughout her life, irrespective of income, employment, family status, or anything else—has a voucher with which she can purchase a health care plan.
- She has invested in and owns that voucher by having paid into its trust fund through dedicated payroll and income taxes whenever she has been employed. Her children and spouse have their own vouchers, and each uses theirs to purchase health care where they want, with dignity, and on the same footing as any other American.
- She has a choice of several different and competitive systems of care at which to redeem that voucher. Each system of care is regulated and has simple and clearly published quality scores for the medical care it provides. She can make her choice based on those objective scores, on convenience, on the presence of the doctor she prefers, on extra services offered, or any other reason she chooses.

- She is free to purchase any additional care or convenience she wants, either as an add-on by her system of care or through external organizations. She can do this herself, or it can be a benefit provided her by her employer, her union, or the state or local government where she lives.
- She has the comfort of knowing that her medical care is taking place in a system with strong and independent audits of its quality.
- The health care system she has become a part of now has strong incentives properly aligned to create value for her: to provide the highest quality services they possibly can with the resources available.

This result is the health care system we've been seeking: universal, fair, high quality, reasonable in its cost, honestly paid for, uniquely American.

13

Twenty Years Later

. . . in which we do a final thought experiment and look into the future to see how our creation has turned out.

One of the rules we all learn about writing is "show, don't tell." Because I've tried to present some concrete ideas about how we might improve the way our health care system operates, I've done quite a bit of "telling" up to this point. I've tried to reimagine our health care system and in doing so have inevitably talked in terms of large ideas: Red Books and systems of care and fairness. I've tried to keep the logic simple and grounded, but when the universe is hundreds of millions of people and trillions of dollars, generalizations and abstractions are inevitable. Let's conclude now with a final thought experiment: let's apply these ideas to some concrete organizations and a patient, imagine ourselves in the future, and try to envision what might have happened. It's now 2030.

Hospitals

America's hospitals have been the big institutional winners. This isn't really surprising, as our new system was built around the concept of tightly integrated systems of care. When we began our new reform, modern hospitals around the country already represented the high-water marks of organization and integration in our health care system. They had the underpinnings of financial strength, systems and management expertise to start, and the least distance to cover to become true systems of care. They were natural nuclei for the new organizations that would be needed.

What repeatedly happened around the country was that one or two of the major hospitals in the central city of the IHSA stepped forward and set up systems of care around their institution. They did this for different reasons: some of them for defensive purposes, to preserve their independence and position, and others as a natural next phase in their growth and an extension of their mission. Everywhere, there were many difficulties in making all the changes that were necessary, but successful modern hospitals brought more assets to the problem than any other institutions.

Here in my home in Nashville, three of the big hospital organizations set up systems of care. Early in our journey, we took a trip to the ninth floor of one of them—Vanderbilt University Medical Center—and so here, a quarter century later, let's revisit and see what has happened.

When the new system was put in place, there was a great deal of internal discussion at Vanderbilt about the future of the institution in this new world. A number of the older and most influential faculty members argued that the medical center needed to remain primarily a specialty hospital, with a focus on research and teaching. They argued that there would always be strong demand for those services and that the Vanderbilt name and reputation would allow it to continue to charge a premium price and thereby benefit the employees and the institution.

However, there was also a strong group of both faculty members and the management of the university that believed they needed to expand and reorganize to become a system of care. Their argument was that if the reality was that the American medical care system was going to be built around integrated systems of care, then Vanderbilt needed to be on the front lines of making them work. They had the professional expertise to do so in a way that honored the ethics of the medical professions. This latter argument carried the day, and while Vanderbilt retained a strong research and teaching program, it committed its delivery system to the system of care concept.

When they sat back and took stock, it was clear that the biggest shortcoming in the delivery system was the lack of primary care capacity. They had long had a strong nursing program, and it rose to the occasion by both expanding the training and finding innovative ways to best use the services of nurse practitioners. That led to a much deeper and more efficient system of primary care, which they found essential in achieving the best quality scores. They evolved a very successful layered system, with nurse practitioners and family practitioners on the front lines, backed up by more specialized professional disciplines as the needs arose.

One of the inevitable results of the standards movement in health care—the Red Book—was the clear need for additional research in a number of areas. Vanderbilt beefed up its medical research capability, and committed substantial additional resources to both research in the effectiveness of various treatments and research in the basic sciences as well. The standards movement quickly made clear that the medical science around numerous mental health diagnoses was in a bad state, and Vanderbilt built a leadership position in this field. It also continued conducting research successfully in some of the areas where it had traditional strength.

The investments that had been made over the years in information system technology in both the hospital and the faculty practice program gave them a strong head start. There was now a real need for sophistication in organizing and monitoring medical care and they were well prepared. In fact, looking back, Vanderbilt attributes their success to having been ready with many of the building blocks of well-organized medical care already in place. This included more than just information systems. They had physicians who were comfortable practicing in an organized environment and a complex and well-run hospital as the centerpiece. They have learned to run a tight system, and as a result, their quality scores have been consistently tops in their region and they've acquired the cachet of a Mayo or Cleveland Clinic. Right now, there's a waiting list for membership in their system of care, and they are in the process of making the business and professional decision as to whether to expand their capacity or continue as they are.

There had been some difficulties. At the outset, they adopted the salaried approach to physician compensation that was in vogue at the time. However, they found that in their particular setting this model resulted in problems with productivity; too many of their physicians didn't work hard enough. About five years ago, they adopted a hybrid approach to compensation, with providers getting a base salary with considerable bonuses depending on both productivity and quality scores. This appears to be working much better, although everyone at the institution expects this issue to be a continuing work in progress for years to come.

The most serious difficulty, however, and one that is not yet completely solved, has been the integration of community-based medical care into the Vanderbilt system. They were, as all systems of care are, required to offer their services over an extended area that included other communities and rural areas in Tennessee and also parts of Kentucky and Alabama. They found in doing so a cultural divide that was difficult to bridge. Especially in the beginning, the academicians at Vanderbilt tended to look down on the providers in small towns and, in turn, those providers resented Vanderbilt's involvement and resisted their attempts to organize care. They were, however, bound together and neither party could just walk away: Vanderbilt had patients in these counties and needed the providers; the providers had to deal with systems of care to get paid.

In a few small communities with limited numbers of providers, Vanderbilt has given up for the time being, and is still paying for medical care on a carefully negotiated and monitored fee-for-service basis. It's concentrating on bringing information technology to bear, in effect resurrecting the payment strategy advocated by reformers back in 2009. The difference, however, was that there were now serious consequences for failure to control costs. Conversely, their greatest successes have been in a number of communities where they have associated with a local community hospital and taken advantage of what was in effect a localized subsystem of care.

In addition to their own successful and competitive system of care, they also enjoy a vigorous referral business from other systems that find it advantageous to buy, rather than build, some kinds of specialty care. While there was initially reluctance by some of their competitors to use them, Vanderbilt has overcome this with quality scores that are reliably high and the perception by patients that it is the blue-chip provider for many life-threatening illnesses. One competitor has even started using the access to Vanderbilt as a marketing tool: their sales strategy is to tout their own convenience and accessibility for routine care, but offer the expertise of Vanderbilt for complex problems.

Vanderbilt regards teaching as its core mission, and is extremely proud of an unanticipated bonus of its decision to embrace the system of care concept. Students who train at the medical and nursing schools or in the residency programs are in exceptionally high demand when they leave, as other systems of care place a high premium on graduates with experience and expertise in this new environment. Vanderbilt has been a winner all around, and their success has been echoed repeatedly across the country where there have been other well-run and integrated hospitals that have chosen to be cores of a complete system of care.

It hasn't been only the big-city regional institutions that have prospered: some of the very best success stories have been with community-based hospitals. Because of their smaller size, they were more nimble in responding to the changes. Their longstanding local presence and community involvement had built up a large reservoir of experience with their citizens, who were far more willing to trust themselves to a system organized by their local hospital than to one from outside the community. In one smaller Tennessee city, for example, a local community set up its own "mini" system of care, bringing in the local medical community as participants and offering itself to all the systems of care as an easy and effective solution to delivering care in the local service area. Their arrangements allowed them to invest, in a variety of ways, in better and more convenient care without having to spend large amounts on underutilized and expensive medical equipment; they provided an agreed-upon range of services; and they referred their patients to the central system of care when that was needed. This model has been repeated many times across the country, and the communities in which this has taken place have some of the greatest satisfaction with the new system that exists anywhere.

Blue Cross

Blue Cross Blue Shield programs have had a harder time of it, but in the end have emerged strong and competitive. They've continued to operate as more open systems, providing medical care primarily through relationships with various community-based providers rather than their own facilities. What has emerged across most of the country is a very competitive battle between highly integrated systems of care such as those centered on hospitals and those that rely more on coordinating a larger number of smaller providers.

At the outset, Blue Cross plans typically had too much invested in traditional approaches to health insurance to contemplate abandoning it willingly. Because of their strong provider base and financial strength, they were for the most part able to quickly qualify as systems of care. They also typically made the decision to continue with an underlying fee-for-service reimbursement system but began experimenting with variations such as bundling payments and various "pay for performance" strategies. In doing so, their calculation was that their potential members would strongly prefer an open system with a wide choice of physicians and hospitals and they could control their costs through careful management and payment incentives to providers.

This was fairly easy to do at first. The voucher system had been set up to minimize dislocations at the outset. In fact, for the first three or four years, all of the traditional insurers fared reasonably well. While the amount they received from the vouchers was capped, there was enough low-hanging fruit to allow them to continue on a traditional path. By the end of the third full year, there were already political figures and commentators who were advocating throwing out the whole reform, saying that the traditional system had shown it could respond and we should back government out of the picture.

It varied from place to place, but it was around the fourth year that the wheels started to come off the strategy. The capping of the vouchers kept a relentless downward pressure on costs and the traditional insurance model was not up to the task. While physicians, for example, were willing to consider simplified approaches to payment, they operated from an underlying assumption that their total income would be maintained and they balked at arrangements that were constraining it. Furthermore, the much more loosely organized model that they were depending upon had difficulties with keeping its quality scores competitive—there was far too much business-as-usual in their delivery systems. City after city had hospital-based systems whose quality scores were in the low eighties and growing. They achieved those scores in a variety of ways, but one important one was simply eliminating providers who were unable or unwilling to practice the kind of evidence-based medicine that was now required. In the more open systems that Blue Cross employed, the providers were far more independent. The result was that in region after region, the Blue Cross systems had quality scores that were ten and fifteen points lower than the more integrated systems, and people started to take notice.

As the pressures mounted, Blue Cross tried the time-tested strategy of using their political clout to get Congress to pay them more. About six years into the new system, they proposed legislation that would increase the voucher amounts for patients who were participating with what they called "traditional community" providers. By this, they meant an open system of local physicians, hospitals, pharmacies, and the like who were still being paid in a traditional fee-for-service model. They ran TV ads, including one called "Yesterday," with a kindly old country doctor telling about how he used to help families. Now they just wanted him to be a cog in a big organization in the name of saving money. This might have been successful in the past, but by this point there was an extensive set of very well-publicized quality scores, and the public took note of the noticeably higher scores of the more tightly integrated systems. Quality of care was being measured and made public in a way that the people could understand and relate to. Public sentiment settled on the common sense position that we shouldn't pay more for lower quality.

Blue Cross plans found themselves with survival at stake and they survived and ultimately prospered by returning to its roots. Blue Cross plans had been founded in the early decades of the twentieth century, not simply as insurance companies, but more fundamentally as a solution to the growing problem of financing hospital care. They had adopted an insurance reimbursement model at the time, but it was a strategy and not the underlying goal of the organization. Faced with some real evidence that the payment model they used had become obsolete, and that clinging to it could cost them their existence, they elected to return to their roots and rethink how they were paying for care. There was considerable public sympathy for what they were trying to do, and while they didn't convince Congress to change the payment amounts, they did convince them to provide substantial grants to their member providers to assist them with a transition. The rationale for this was a reasonable one: to ensure that there was a competitive market place in the ways that health care would be delivered.

The solution for Blue Cross was a massive investment in information technology. They required all their providers to use that technology or a compatible one of their own choosing. In other words, a physician group, for example, as a condition of participating in the Blue Cross delivery system, had to have an integrated medical information system that could communicate with Blue Cross in real time. Blue Cross was willing to provide such a system, or providers could use their own as long as the capabilities were there. Those systems became real-time tools in the physician offices in the practice of medicine. The information systems reminded physicians—while the patient was still present—of current standards, suggested options, and flagged actions that were contrary to best practices or unnecessary. Where there were providers whose expertise was questionable or out-of-date, the information systems provided assistance and a check on mistakes that kept them productive and safe.

The information systems also provided a way for the system of care itself to set and enforce standards that helped them navigate the tension of cost and quality that was needed. Systems of care could set policies as to under what circumstances certain drugs were prescribed or tests ordered. While they almost universally left the final decisions in the hands of the medical professional, they found that asking providers to provide a level of justification for actions outside of or contrary to standards was both a substantial cost-saving device and improved quality as well. It also allowed for the review of some particularly important or expensive decisions by experts. Where some additional approvals had long been a part of the payment system, it was transformed from a crude tool designed largely to place barriers in the way of some services into a true quality and cost control measure.

Some of the original third-party payers weren't able to change and went out of business. But many Blue Cross plans and their commercial insurance cousins were so successful in this effort—it was what should have been done a generation ago—that they've prospered. The successful ones are those who abandoned the insurance role and reinvented themselves as health care providers, but ones who operated primarily through contracts with independent suppliers. They use a variety of contractual arrangements to accomplish this and these arrangements are worked out on the fine scale of individual systems of care and specific providers rather than any national model. For that reason, they're much richer in their variety and inventiveness, and better tailored to specific communities and situations.

Physicians

The practice of medicine has changed, and inevitably some physicians have liked the changes and prospered, while others have not.

One unexpected development was that the growing trend toward more and larger group practices was reversed. The combination of simpler and less costly payment systems, powerful information systems, and the assumption of various risks such as malpractice by the system of care made the practice of medicine in small groups and even solo practices more practical and attractive. There were providers—both physicians and nurse practitioners—who now found it practical and attractive to live and work in smaller communities, and the decades of decline in the availability of rural health services was reversed. The combination of primary care providers, some specialists, and a layer of hospital services in smaller communities, working in combination with more expensive and specialized ones in the central urban areas, became an attractive one for everyone involved.

One of the initial responses of physicians in some communities was to present a united front to the systems of care and attempt to keep rates high and a traditional fee-for-service system in place. In some cases groups legally consolidated to produce a practical monopoly in the marketplace. In most cities, there were specialties and subspecialties that were already consolidated in a single group and able to use that power in their negotiations with systems of care (just as they had done before with private insurers). These produced some of the most heated and divisive battles, but resolution of those, while painful, was exactly the kind of change that the health care system needed.

Looking back on this transition, it worked best in areas where there was a rough parity in the strength of systems of care and the provider community. In Nashville, there were five systems of care, a moderately consolidated physician community, and a large number of smaller rural communities with single hospitals and limited numbers of physicians. With this mix, there was no party that could dominate the negotiation, most parties saw that their interests lay in working out accommodations, and the transition was sometimes painful, but in the end quite successful.

The problems occurred where the strengths were not comparable. In some areas, there was a single essential provider—typically a large hospital system or a children's hospital—that was necessary to provide health care. There were several systems of care, and the essential provider didn't need them all, and so could divide and conquer. There were also areas that were the mirror image of this. With a dominant system of care and a divided provider community. In these cases it was the system of care in a position to divide and conquer. In the end, these were resolved as monopolies frequently are—too much greed makes alternatives possible.

A few systems of care that were unable to come to terms with powerful providers looked elsewhere. In both the for-profit and nonprofit hospital industry, for example, there was an abundance of private capital available and well-respected parties willing to come to a community and build a hospital in return for long-term contracts with systems of care. In some areas this happened, in others the credible threat was all that was needed.

Similarly, where there was a system of care that was dominant and a fragmented provider community, groups of providers formed organizations to approach other systems of care with the offer of long-term contracts if they would come to the providers' area. The immediate availability of a broad and respected provider base made entry into the new market an attractive investment. Again, in some places this happened, in others the threat was enough. For both systems of care and providers, as always, the ones that bought a short-term peace just faced the problem again. Those that held out for long-term arrangements with multiyear advance notice of terminations created a stable environment and got on with the business of providing health care to their patients.

While there was a resurgence in the attractiveness and viability of smaller practices, there were many large multispecialty groups that prospered as well. They were large enough to have the management systems to operate efficiently and their financial capability made them more flexible in the ways in which they could contract. Most of them preferred to remain independent of any particular system of care and contract with a number of them who operated in their service area. The systems of care found these groups very attractive. They delivered high quality care at competitive costs and the groups often became respected brands in their area in their own right. They were well positioned to prosper in the system of incentives that the nation's new approach to health care had put in place. They would reliably deliver high quality scores and their brand attracted patients. As a result, they commanded premium prices, their practitioners did well financially, and the group was therefore quick to deal with practitioners who lowered quality scores or increased costs.

Winners

Change of this magnitude under any circumstances would create a great many opportunities, and the changes in the organization and financing of the health care system proved a particularly rich field. Some of the winners were obvious in advance. Information systems topped the list, and nearly all of the managerial disciplines that modern organizations use—human resources, recruiting, marketing, financial analysis, legal, professional development—were suddenly in demand by both systems of care and providers who had to reorganize how they worked around principles of quality and cost control.

The biggest winners were those organizations—some entrepreneurial and some established—who could offer systems of care better and less expensive ways to deliver patient care. Services such as telephone and Internet advice and follow-up exploded in volume and added further depth to the primary care system at lower cost. Data mining and analysis helped systems of care understand better their own operation and focus on areas that were problematical or offered the best return for additional investment. There were relatively few start-up organizations that entered the business of actually starting and operating systems of care. The capital and scale required meant that existing organizations dominated that field. But there were a great many who provided innovative services to them and prospered. One venture-funded start-up, for example, developed a model for managing diabetes and created a large and successful business building highly regarded specialized clinics around the country. These would contract to accept a fixed payment from the system of care for patients who voluntarily chose them. They became expert in this area, created excellent quality scores, and allowed the system of care to better control its costs for diabetic patients. Another start-up became highly proficient in performing independent quality assessments. Systems of care used them to find problems early and not be blindsided by audit results.

Patients who belonged to systems of care for their basic needs were free to expand their purchase of health care, and a number of businesses sought to offer add-on products through the system of care for an additional price. One particularly successful start-up offered house calls by nurse practitioners for an additional premium and fee, and is growing steadily across the country, with many imitators.

Losers

There were also, of course, plenty of losers, as in any competitive economic system. The cost and quality of health care had suffered for decades from those who—making perfectly rational business decisions in the system that existed—created demand for expensive products and services that were in excess of what was medically required. They took advantage of the fact that the patient had limited information and little or no stake in paying for the services.

Pharmaceutical companies were put under a great deal of pressure by the new system and their profits declined. The business model of setting high prices on drugs and marketing them aggressively to physicians and sometimes directly to patients quickly came to an end. The systems of care had to control their costs and began to broadly use generics and less-expensive branded pharmaceuticals where they would do the job satisfactorily. There was now a strong reason to choose pharmaceuticals based on efficacy and cost. Systems of care were now able to negotiate with the pharmaceutical companies, and where different companies had drugs with similar therapeutic effects, make them compete on price. Pharmaceutical research became more directed at producing drugs that could command a higher price because of their uncontested efficacy. The industry continued as a viable and profitable one, but the glory days of the 1990s and 2000s were over.

While many physicians have done very well in the new system, with more money available for their professional services as less is spent on unneeded things, there are some whose incomes have declined substantially under the new system. Surgeons who earned seven-figure incomes doing spinal fusions and those who did large numbers of aggressive cardiac procedures—stents, for example—were among those who saw their practices decline substantially, and were forced to broaden their patient base. Physicians and institutions that bought expensive technology such as imaging equipment and overused it found that their profit center was cut off.

There had been a number of provider organizations that had developed to extract profitable segments of business from existing providers. This included some specialty hospitals, for example, and some of the ambulatory surgery centers. Life has been difficult for them this past decade, with many of them going out of business or merging with other providers. Pharmacies, likewise, had to change their business model, as the mix and profitability of the drugs they dispensed changed as alternative ways of delivering those drugs to the patient grew. Where a simple prescription for an acute illness—an antibiotic, for example—was needed, it was often simply given out in the doctor's office, saving money, time, and gas for the patient. While there were losers in these changes, many of the people and organizations involved quickly found other ways of participating in the health care system that were more productive and better for the patient.

Patients

Of course, none of this change would make any sense if patients themselves were not the ultimate beneficiary. There was a lot of anxiety in the earliest years, but that rapidly subsided as the systems of care and their providers worked out the rough spots and began working together. Patients by the tens of millions are getting better health care now, but we'll end our journey with the story of just one.

Back in the present, several chapters ago, we stood on the ninth floor of the Vanderbilt Medical Center and looked out over Edgehill, a poor inner-city neighborhood in Nashville. At another time, I had been in that Edgehill neighborhood and met a young woman I'll call Joan, who was pregnant and, who had health insurance through the Medicaid program, but who was not getting her prenatal checkups. Vanderbilt wasn't that far physically from where she lived in public housing, but there was an enormous cultural distance, and the bustle, the white coats, and the unfamiliarity of the place was like another planet to her. In her neighborhood, there were well-meaning young people with their grant funding—that's what I was there to see—commuting into the neighborhood to encourage her and others like her to get that prenatal care.

She eventually had a little girl, right there at Vanderbilt, through the emergency room. The baby was born before she reached full term and was one of the low-birth-weight babies that contributed to the terrible health care statistics in the area. Vanderbilt did a great job in their neonatal intensive care unit, and after an expensive stay, the baby was stabilized and Joan took her home. I don't know what she named that little girl, but I'll call her Jill. I hope that Jill will grow up, move out of the projects, and get a college education and a good job. But she might not, and while there might be many reasons for that, one of them might be some of the effects of the way in which she was born. It can't be helpful to start out in this world too small, on a respirator, and in an incubator instead of a mother's arms.

Let's now return to our future, which is about twenty years after my visit. Jill is unfortunately still there in Edgehill, and now she's pregnant herself. Once again, her health care challenges are not an issue of payment. Jill, like her mother, has excellent coverage. For our new health care system to have meaning it should make the way things work for Jill better than the old system did for her mom.

It does. Jill became part of the Vanderbilt system of care at an early age. What that meant was that a large, powerful, financially

strong institution had a direct economic and professional interest in seeing that all her health care was provided properly. Their
strong incentive was to ensure that all of the health care she needed
was available and professionally delivered and not just to be there
for one highly professional, heroic, and last-minute intervention.
If Jill had a premature, low-birth-weight baby, that baby wouldn't
be a revenue generator, it would be a major economic loss. That
outcome would hurt the Vanderbilt system of care's quality scores,
rather than a professionally excellent stay in the hospital would
help them.

Vanderbilt, because of its location, had a large number of Jills
in their system of care. In addition to their evident professional
concern, they were very aware of the risks these women presented
to both their quality scores and the economics of their institution.
So they reached out and put a clinic right in the Edgehill neighborhood that was directly tied to Vanderbilt. They used their information systems to keep track of Jill and stay in contact with her.
They made sure she was getting medical care herself, and when she
became pregnant, they upped their attention level to make sure she
was healthy and got the prenatal care she needed. They helped educate Jill on what she had to do to have a healthy baby. They were
innovative about how they did these things, because they cared
about and had a real stake in the results. They weren't executing a
grant contract, they were risking their own money.

Local government in Nashville had appropriated money to add
to the health care voucher amount for additional nonmedical services for pregnant women in some of the city's poorer areas. They
entered into an agreement with Vanderbilt to provide parenting
assistance both before and after the birth of Jill's baby. This was a
natural and efficient way to provide this additional nonhealth-care
support.

Much of this care had been available in some form for a long time.
The difference now was that again, there was a strong institution

with a direct, compelling economic and professional interest when it came to Jill as an individual. They were responsible for all of her health care and they were innovative and focused about how they went about fulfilling that responsibility. What counted were results for Jill and not the bill to Medicaid or the contractual terms of a grant.

Finally, Jill had her baby, another little girl. She was born healthy and normal, the cost to the medical care system was modest. Jill's daughter was far better served by America's medical care system that she and her mother had been.

America

From our vantage point in the future, the preceding twenty years have been a good time in America. It had taken a serious crisis to get the president and Congress to finally act and create a truly sustainable and high quality health care system. Once the new system was underway, however, it became clear that we were now genuinely controlling costs and the new system was liked by our citizens. That gave everyone the confidence to take the final steps to permanently stabilize the whole social insurance system in America—to make sure we never slipped back into the dangerous hole that had almost bankrupted us. Today, our health care costs are actually lower than those in some other nations, but the medical care our citizens receive is once again the best in the world. It's been painful, we've had a backslide or two along the way, but we've done it.

Social insurance programs weren't foreseen by our nation's founders, but if those founders were able to return today and visit our complex and interconnected society, they would understand them. They would see them as a confirmation of their dream for their new country—a people and a system of government that would always respond to the challenges and possibilities just as they had done.

They'd see social insurance as the latest way in which we have been able to change and adapt as a free people. They wouldn't be too troubled by the struggles of the last part of the twentieth century and first part of the twenty-first in making it work. They'd be proud, instead, of the final result, of how we eventually brought this responsibility smoothly into the fabric of our nation.

This year, Congress passed a simple constitutional amendment to formally recognize this new role for our democracy and permanently ensure that we would always handle it safely and well. It reads:

Twenty-seventh amendment (social insurance trust funds)

1. Any social insurance program shall operate only as a trust fund whose finances are kept separate and distinct from those of general government.
2. The receipts of each trust fund shall come from sources determined by Congress and transmitted directly to the trust fund. Any additional general appropriation by Congress to the trust fund shall require a 3/5 roll call vote of Congress directly on that subject.
3. Prior to each fiscal year, for each such trust fund, Congress shall adopt a statement of expected receipts and outlays for each of the following twenty years in which total outlays over the period do not exceed total receipts.
4. Each trust fund may borrow to meet its obligations and must include interest and complete repayment of principal within twenty years in its anticipated outlays.
5. Congress shall have the power to enforce this article by appropriate legislation.
6. This article shall take effect for the fifth fiscal year after its ratification.

There is strong national support for this, and we all expect it to be ratified by thirty-eight states in the next three or four years.

America has not only fixed its health care, it's built a responsive and uniquely American system. We've become the envy of the world for the dignity, efficiency and the quality of our medical care. Our health care costs and our deficits are under control. Other countries now look to America for inspiration in this sphere of life as well. Once again, Americans have proven that we can "promote the general welfare and secure the blessings of liberty to ourselves and our posterity." Which is as it should be.

Epilogue

I was flying back to Nashville not long ago, it was well into the evening, almost night, and I was sitting alone with the lights dimmed, looking out the window. I could still just see the fields, the roads, and now the lights of the towns and farms of Tennessee. In the evening haze, they seemed insubstantial against the vast darkening land. I felt I could look beneath these superficial markings and still glimpse the original America of dark forests and rivers and mountains, when it was a new land that God had given us on which to build a nation. I thought it would have been a wonderful thing to have lived then, to have been one of those pioneers, and to have awoken each morning and felt the miracle of a fresh new world and its promise of an unlimited future.

That thought had no more than taken form when I realized the truth: America still is that land. Our world is still young and we only need, when the way seems obscured, to reach inside and re-attach ourselves to the dream that graces our nation.

Sitting there, looking out that airplane window at the land growing dark below, I thought about the work that it took those first pioneers to carve a new life out of this land. Those families had to clear fields, dig wells, plant crops. And the most important task of all: before the harvest was in, they had to raise a barn. Building a barn wasn't something that a family could do alone, so when the time came, they asked their neighbors for help, and everyone came together for a barn raising. This was a community responsibility.

Imagine that barn raising with me for a moment: a wide open field surrounded by forest. The sky is just getting light, but men and women are coming together, crossing the field, from north and south and east and west. Soon you can hear the saws, and the hammers, and voices and shouts. By the time the sun is on the field, you can see the framework—men and women at the foundation, on ladders, a few men climbing along the main beam, nailing the rafters.

These were fiercely independent people, these pioneers, but when they raised a barn, they did something special. Pioneers were just as human as we are today: they had grudges, agendas, and many different beliefs about what values the world they were creating should embrace. But on that day, they put aside their disagreements and they postponed other projects. They didn't have the luxury of comfortable lives with free-ranging egos. They lived in a dangerous world, and knew there were times simply to do what was needed and do it together. They gathered in that field, got to work, and the sun came up the next morning on a new barn.

I like to imagine that pioneer family arising on the day that followed and looking out on their new barn. And I believe that as they stood there—still deeply self-reliant—they saw in that barn both their own future and a deep truth: that there are times when asking and accepting the help of their neighbors doesn't diminish independence, it strengthens it. Our nation has always prized individual freedom and I pray it always will. But the world grows and changes, and each generation finds new barns to be built, new things—a sensible approach to health care among them—that truly are and must be a community responsibility. When we accept that responsibility, we don't diminish individual freedom, we strengthen and renew it.

In 1791, Thomas Paine wrote in the *Rights of Man,* "A little matter will move a party, but it must be something great that moves a nation." I appeal to our president: with health care, you've moved a party, now move a nation. However you choose to proceed, you are an extraordinarily gifted man and we need your leadership.

We have to face this problem. The idea of America is far grander than a self-indulgent nation, paralyzed, spiraling ever deeper into debt until our bankers finally call a halt.

I looked out the window of that airplane over Tennessee and thought: in America God gave us an opportunity, not a guarantee. The threats to the dream we've inherited change over the years, but this is still a dangerous land. The miracle is that we're still young and our vision of an unlimited future still strong. Right now, we need to build some barns.

Acknowledgments

While this book obviously represents a very personal view of health care and I take full responsibility for its contents, I want to acknowledge a few of the many people whose counsel and ideas have helped me a great deal in developing these thoughts and communicating them.

First, a small group from Vanderbilt University met with me a number of times in the summer and fall of 2009 to help with research and to clarify my thinking. Their knowledge of health care, quick intelligence, and willingness to challenge ideas made these meetings some of the most rewarding times I have ever spent exploring any subject. The group was led by M. Kathleen Figaro, M.D., and included Lara Bratcher, M.D., Philip Ciampa, M.D., and Bradford Cayer and Jesse Cuthrell, both students at the time at the Owen Graduate School of Management.

Larry Van Horn, an associate professor at the Owen Graduate School of Management, was instrumental in making my connection to this group, was willing to discuss at length the economics of health care, and offered numerous constructive suggestions on an early draft of the book.

Darin Gordon, Tennessee's Medicaid director, is extraordinarily knowledgeable about the organization and delivery of health care, and he and his medical director, Wendy Long, M.D., M.P.H., contributed a great deal to bringing my 1980's knowledge of the medical care system into the twenty-first century. (All on their own time.)

Vivian Riefberg is a friend, advisor on all health care matters, a senior partner in McKinsey & Company's Washington, D.C. office where she leads the health care practice, and the person who probably *should* have written this book.

Will Pinkston, a former journalist for the Nashville *Tennessean* and *The Wall Street Journal* and a senior staff member in my office, read a draft and offered excellent suggestions on how to improve the clarity of my presentation.

Vicky Gregg, the president and CEO of Blue Cross/Blue Shield of Tennessee, and now the Chair of AHIP (America's Health Insurance Plans), has long been very generous to me with her deep knowledge of the health insurance industry and introduced me to several people around the nation who were willing to talk with me about issues in that field.

Karl Van Devender, M.D., is my doctor and helped me understand how a modern multispecialty practice works; Brian Haile, the deputy director of Benefits Administration for the State of Tennessee is my resident expert on health insurance Exchanges.

While I've had no communication with any of them in regard to these ideas or this book, some of the thoughts have obvious roots in the work over the past decades of Alain Enthoven, Marriner S. Eccles professor of public and private management, Emeritus at Stanford University, particularly in his work on integrated delivery systems and "managed competition"; of Uwe Reinhardt, James Madison professor of political economy at Princeton University, particularly his work on tying physician payment to quality measures; and of Paul Starr, professor of sociology and public affairs, Princeton University, whose 1984 book, *The Social Transformation of American Medicine,* first stimulated my thinking about the public policy dimensions of health care.

Lydia Peelle knows nothing about health care whatsoever, but is my former speechwriter and a published, accomplished, and upcoming writer of fiction. She provided the essential advice that every would-be author needs to hear from someone: "Stop talking about it, sit down at your desk, and actually put down one word. Repeat."

Most of all, I want to acknowledge and thank my wife, Andrea Conte, a nurse. I hope that everything I've written honors her compassion for those less fortunate than she and her belief that all medical care is for the benefit of patients and not providers.